GLUTEN-FREE RECIPES IN 30 MINUTES

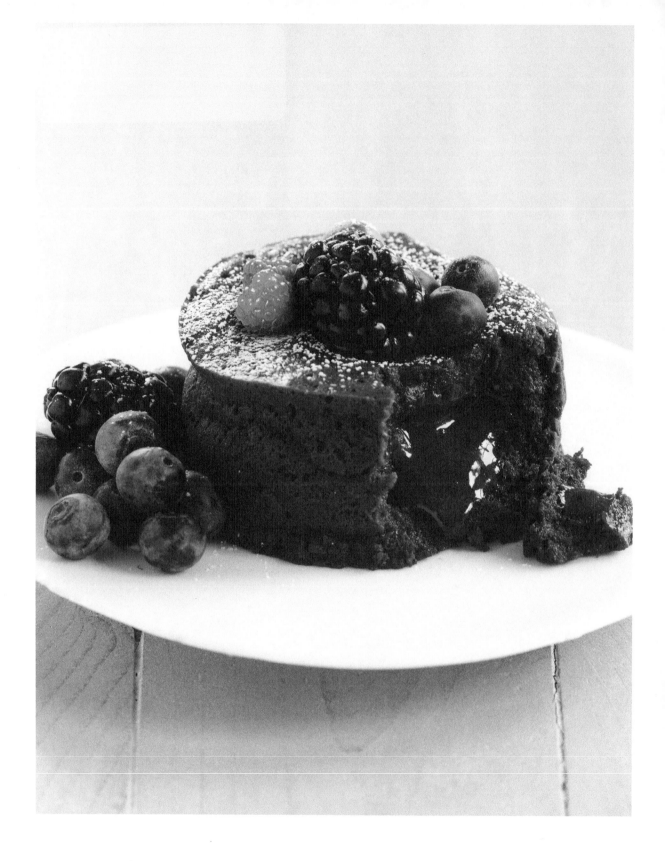

GLUTEN-FREE
RECIPES IN
30 MINUTES

*A Gluten-Free Cookbook
with 137 Quick & Easy Recipes
Prepared in 30 Minutes*

**SHASTA
PRESS**

CONTENTS

6

Appetizers and Snacks   79

7

Salads   105

8

Soups, Stews, and Chilies   117

9

Vegetarian Entrées   131

10
Fish, Seafood, and Meat Entrées 147

11
Desserts 171

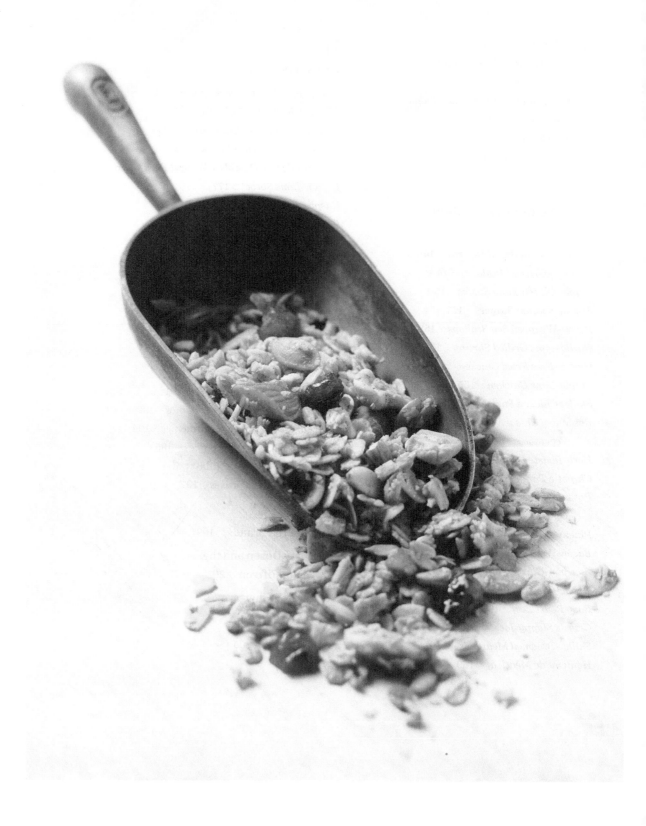

INTRODUCTION

Eliminating gluten from your diet can offer significant health benefits. But it is no small undertaking. If you are trying for the first time to eliminate gluten from your diet, you may well be in a bit of a panic. Most of us eat gluten for breakfast, lunch, and dinner as well as for snacks and dessert. You may be wondering what is left for you to eat. Take comfort in the fact that the gluten-free way of life has become much more common over the past decade or so, and many, many people have traveled this road before you. They have discovered that you can eat well and thoroughly enjoy your food while still eliminating gluten. This book will show you how to follow in their footsteps.

In this book, you'll find information that will help you adopt a gluten-free life-style as easily and painlessly as possible. You'll gain an understanding of what gluten is. You'll learn which foods contain gluten and how to avoid them. You'll also learn the cooking techniques necessary and master the tools you'll need to go gluten-free, including dozens of fantastic recipes for delicious, healthy, budget-friendly, and family-friendly foods that you'll be able to enjoy.

While many gluten-free cookbooks and websites rely on complicated or time-consuming cooking techniques and expensive or hard-to-find ingredients, this book provides recipes that are quick and easy and use ingredients that are both affordable and easy to find. All the recipes in the book are easy to prepare, and none will require you to search the ends of the Earth or pawn your prized possessions for special ingredients.

The book is divided into two parts. Part 1 tells you all you need to know to understand the gluten-free diet and get started on making the transition in your own life. It explains what gluten is, why some people cannot eat it, and what the health benefits of eliminating it from your diet are. It also provides a detailed guide to getting started on a gluten-free diet, including lists of foods to eat and foods to avoid, and tips for making the transition as easy as possible. Finally, it offers guidance on what kitchen tools you'll need to stock up on, how to save time while cooking, how to convert standard recipes to be gluten-free, and how to bake gluten-free.

The editors of this book understand that while health is the goal of a gluten-free diet, simple and delicious recipes are the path to success. Part 2 offers more than 120 quick and easy gluten-free recipes prepared in less than 30 minutes. These dishes are a cinch to make, highly nutritious, family-friendly, easy on the budget, and full of flavor. You'll also find time-saving tips, ingredient tips, and cooking tips tucked in with the recipes to make things even easier. With these recipes, you can begin your gluten-free life eating delicious and satisfying meals.

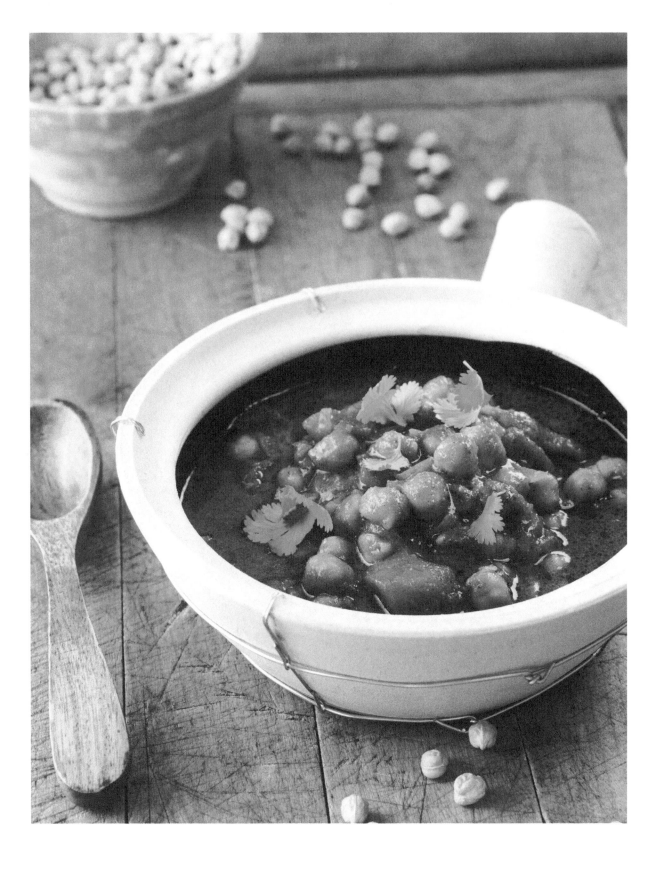

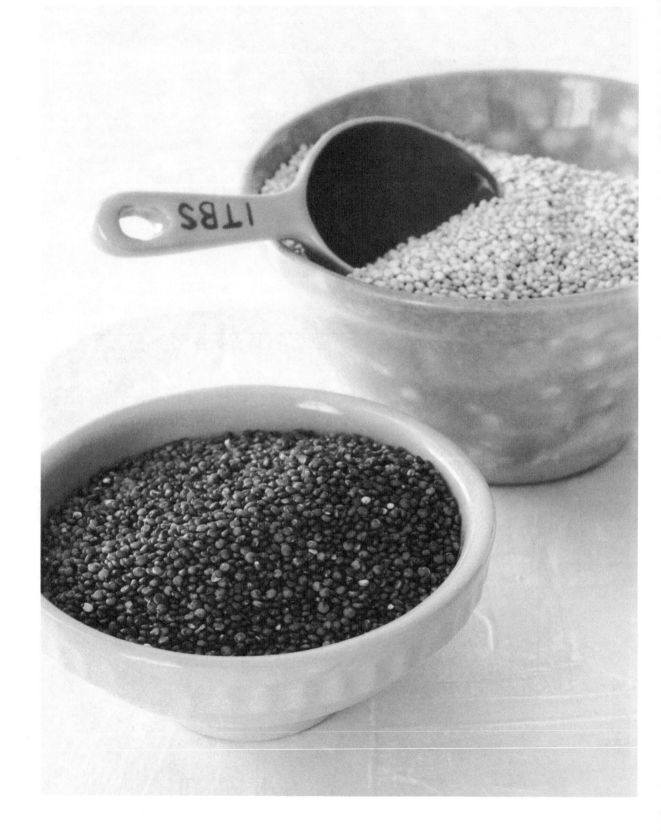

1

The Gluten-Free Diet

A gluten-free diet, at its most basic, is a diet that excludes gluten and all foods that contain gluten, such as wheat, barley, rye, and triticale (a wheat-rye hybrid). The goal of such a diet is to reduce the inflammation that gluten causes in the digestive system of individuals with celiac disease or gluten sensitivity.

If you have a mild gluten sensitivity, you might be able to get away with a little exposure now and then, but for those with serious allergies or immune responses such as celiac disease, any amount of gluten carries an enormous health risk. The true gluten-free diet involves eliminating every speck of gluten from your diet—even the trace amounts that may be present due to cross-contamination (when a gluten-free food comes into contact with gluten), the small amounts of gluten in foods like soy sauce and malt vinegar, and even traces of gluten that may linger in medications or herbal supplements.

The gluten-free diet, then, involves eliminating all foods that obviously contain gluten, such as commercially prepared bread, pasta, cereal, and many snack foods and processed foods. It also involves reading labels and snooping out hidden sources of gluten in foods typically not associated with grains, such as mustard, soy sauce, and chewing gum.

So standard breads, cakes, cookies, and other baked goods; standard soy sauce and tamari sauce as well as foods that contain them; most cereals, including many oat-based cereals; and anything containing any form of wheat, barley, rye, or triticale are all out of the diet.

Right about now, you may be thinking, "Wait, doesn't that cover just about every-thing?" It's true that the modern American diet relies heavily on wheat and other grains that contain gluten, but there are plenty of other types of delicious foods that are entirely gluten-free: Fresh vegetables and fruits, meat, fish, seafood, eggs, nuts, and seeds are all on the gluten-free menu. Plus, there are now loads of gluten-free alternatives to choose from in the supermarket and health food store.

With a bit of research, vigilance, and careful shopping, you can still enjoy most of your favorite foods. Rather than feeling deprived, you will likely find that you feel better than ever because you are eating foods that support and heal your body rather than stimulate it to fight against itself.

Celiac Disease and Gluten Sensitivity

The gluten-free diet is essential to treat and manage celiac disease. Celiac disease is a severe autoimmune disease; sufferers can become extremely ill when they eat even trace amounts of gluten.

When a person who has celiac disease consumes gluten, it triggers an autoimmune reaction, treating the protein as a foreign substance. In addition to attacking the foreign invader, however, the immune system also starts to attack normal tissue, particularly in the lining of the small intestine. This leads to inflammation and other gastrointestinal symptoms. It may also affect the body's ability to absorb nutrients, including vitamins A, D, E, and K, as well as iron, calcium, protein, and fat. Nutritional deficiencies are a fairly common result of celiac disease, leading to other problems, such as osteoporosis, fatigue, delayed growth, and more.

Celiac disease that is not treated can lead to other autoimmune disorders, including type 1 diabetes, multiple sclerosis, anemia, osteoporosis, infertility and miscarriage, neurological conditions such as epilepsy and migraines, and intestinal cancers.

According to the National Foundation for Celiac Awareness, an estimated 1 percent of the US population has celiac disease—although that number may rise because it is also estimated that 83 percent of Americans who have the disease are undiagnosed or misdiagnosed.

Many people who don't have celiac disease have some level of gluten sensitivity or intolerance, also known as non-celiac gluten sensitivity. These people cannot tolerate gluten and have symptoms similar to those with celiac disease, but they do not experience the same intestinal damage seen in people with celiac disease. According to the University of Maryland Center for Celiac Research, gluten sensitivity affects approximately 6 percent of the US population, or 18 million people.

Gluten sensitivity can cause unpleasant symptoms, including gastrointestinal problems (gas, bloating, diarrhea, and/or constipation); fatigue or "brain fog" after consuming gluten; neurological symptoms such as dizziness or loss of balance; hormone imbalances that can lead to premenstrual syndrome (PMS), polycystic ovarian syndrome (PCOS—an imbalance of female sex hormones), or unexplained infertility; migraines; chronic fatigue; fibromyalgia; inflammation and swelling or pain in the joints; and mood disorders such as anxiety, depression, mood swings, or attention deficit disorder.

Get tested before you go gluten-free. If you think you might have a gluten sensitivity or celiac disease—for instance if you've found that when you eat gluten, you develop gastrointestinal symptoms such as diarrhea, cramping, gas, bloating, or constipation— see a doctor and get tested for celiac disease before you eliminate gluten from your diet. This is because after you eliminate gluten from your diet, the diagnostic test might not be able to detect celiac disease, even if you have it.

What Is Gluten?

Gluten is a type of protein found in certain grains, including wheat, barley, rye, and triticale. It is a component of most standard baked goods, and for good reason: It's what gives dough its elasticity and rise and the chewy, spongy texture we crave. Gluten is found in many other processed foods, as well, since manufacturers use these grain products and isolated gluten for consistency, texture, and flavoring in many foods.

To eliminate gluten from your diet, you'll have to go further than eliminating breads, cookies, and cakes. You'll need to learn how to identify gluten in the foods you buy and consume. Any foods that contain wheat, barley, rye, or triticale are obviously off-limits. But some foods you might not expect also contain gluten.

Gluten is in a lot of food products that are not grain-based, such as malt vinegar, soy sauce, many oats and products containing oats, and even some lunch meats, nutritional supplements, and medications. Commercial condiments such as mayonnaise, mustard, barbecue sauce, and ketchup may use gluten as a binder and stabilizer. Tomato sauce and tomato paste often contain gluten, as well. In all these foods, gluten will not be listed on the label.

Other products may be dusted with or processed with flour or made on equipment that is dusted with flour. These include chewing gum, candy bars, and yeast. And wheat may be an additive in everything from ice cream to corn- and rice-based cereals. Gluten can even turn up in household products. Art supplies and household adhesives often contain gluten, as do many cleaning agents and toiletries.

To identify gluten in foods, be sure to read labels carefully. First, look for the obvious—wheat, barley, rye, or triticale. But while products containing wheat must list wheat on their label, be aware that food producers are not required to disclose ingredients that are made from barley or rye. Many food additives, both natural or artificial, contain gluten. Learn what they are and keep that list handy when you're reading labels.

Your best defense is to know what's in the product and how it's made—and you can't always tell that just from reading the label. Contact the manufacturer; there's almost always a phone number and a website on the label. Or else stick with products that are labeled as gluten-free.

Watch out for cross-contamination. Even trace amounts of gluten can be dangerous for someone with celiac disease. If you or someone in your household suffers from celiac, be diligent about avoiding cross-contamination (gluten from one source being transferred to another). Use separate toasters for gluten-free and regular breads. Don't share flour sifters or storage containers between gluten-free foods and grains with gluten. And never dip gluten products into foods—such as hummus, peanut butter, or jam—that will be consumed by those who are gluten-free.

Benefits of a Gluten-Free Diet

If you have celiac disease, the only treatment is a gluten-free diet. Avoiding gluten means avoiding the symptoms that appear when you eat it—and heading off the health risks associated with untreated celiac disease.

If you have an allergy or sensitivity to gluten, the gluten-free diet may offer a variety of health benefits, from improved gastrointestinal health to increased energy levels. For people with a mild to moderate gluten sensitivity, eating a gluten-free diet may improve overall well-being, trigger weight loss, improve digestion, boost energy levels, and improve focus and mental clarity.

Improved Digestive Function

If you suffer from chronic digestive problems, including gas, cramping, diarrhea, or constipation, eliminating gluten from your diet may help. People with some degree of gluten sensitivity can reduce the frequency and severity of these symptoms by going gluten-free.

Improved Mood and Mental Clarity

People suffering from even mild gluten sensitivity may experience headaches, mental fogginess, difficulty focusing, and even depression as their body reacts to gluten by attacking its own tissues and causing inflammation in the nervous system. This can lead to mood disorders such as depression or anxiety. Similarly, gluten interferes with the body's absorption of the protein tryptophan, which is responsible for a general sense of well-being and relaxation. Without tryptophan, a person can experience depressed mood. As a result, eliminating gluten can improve mental clarity and mood.

Increased Energy

Gluten sensitivity can cause inflammation in the digestive tract that interferes with digestion and the absorption of important vitamins and minerals, such as iron, calcium, magnesium, vitamins B12 and D, zinc, folate, niacin, and riboflavin. Deficiency in these nutrients often leads to feelings of fatigue and muscle weakness. For many, eliminating gluten can lead to improved energy levels and increased vigor.

Decreased Joint Pain

Eating gluten can cause an autoimmune reaction in those who are sensitive to it. One common symptom of this reaction is inflammation and pain in the joints, including the hips, knees, and back. Eliminating gluten from the diet can help reduce this joint inflammation and pain.

Weight Loss

There is much debate about how—and even whether—going gluten-free leads to weight loss, but many people do lose weight when they switch to a gluten-free diet. In her article published by the *Huffington Post*, registered dietician Katherine Tallmadge argues that the weight loss is not due to the gluten-free diet but simply due to the fact that going gluten-free limits the foods available, leading you to eat less and lose weight.

According to Dr. Mark Hyman, wheat stimulates the appetite, leading you to eat more than you would if you skipped the wheat. Wheat consumption may also stimulate insulin production, which leads to fat storage. But the fact remains that there is anecdotal data that eliminating gluten from your diet can help you shed some extra pounds. If your decision to go gluten-free is motivated by a desire to lose weight, it is certainly worth a try.

What to Watch Out For

While there are numerous potential benefits of a gluten-free diet, there are some caveats, as well. Sufferers of celiac disease *must* eliminate gluten from their diet to manage their symptoms and keep themselves healthy. Even people with mild gluten sensitivity may find that they feel worlds better after they eliminate the gluten in their diet. But gluten-free is not a cure-all and can't be relied on, by itself, to preserve or promote good health for everyone.

Gluten-Free Doesn't Necessarily Mean Nutritious

A gluten-free diet can be extremely healthy, but that doesn't mean gluten-free foods are necessarily health foods. In fact, many gluten-free substitutes—for breads, bagels, pastas, and the like—are actually less nutritious than the standard versions. That's because the manufacturers often replace whole wheat and other whole grains with less nutritious grains, such as white rice, which contain fewer vitamins, minerals, and other nutrients.

Be Mindful of Calories

Makers of many gluten-free foods replace whole grains—wheat, barley, and rye, for instance—with highly processed grains and then boost the fat and sugar content to make up for the loss in flavor. As a result, these gluten-free products are not only lower in nutrition but also higher in calories—empty calories. Be sure to read nutrition labels and eat a balanced diet.

Don't Forget the Fiber

Since white rice and other highly processed grains are often used as substitutes for whole grains, gluten-free products are often much lower in fiber than the originals. When going gluten-free, be sure to eat a diet that is rich in whole, high-fiber foods like beans and whole (gluten-free) grains like quinoa, brown rice, and amaranth.

Gluten-Free Is Not a Magic Weight-Loss Bullet

Many people switch to a gluten-free diet to lose weight, but it's not uncommon for people to gain weight when going gluten-free. This is likely due to the fact that many newly gluten-free dieters choose gluten-free replacements for their favorite foods, such as breads, bagels, crackers, pasta, and cookies. While these foods may be of limited nutritional value to begin with, the gluten-free versions are often even less nutritious but higher in calories. As a result, many gluten-free foods are lower in vitamins and minerals and higher in carbohydrates, fat, and calories than their counterparts with gluten. And that is not a recipe for weight loss.

Watch Your Wallet

The gluten-free product market has expanded exponentially in recent years. These days, just about every supermarket has a section devoted to gluten-free foods, from pasta, crackers, and soy sauce to cereals, cookies, and cakes. Be warned that gluten-free products are generally significantly more expensive than the foods they are meant to replace. Learn to cook gluten-free versions of your favorite foods at home, or better yet, stick to whole foods like fresh fruits and vegetables, beans and legumes, nuts and seeds, and meat, poultry, and fish.

Foods to Enjoy

Right about now, you might be feeling a little depressed. The list of foods you have to give up to embrace a gluten-free lifestyle is long and surely contains some of your favorites. The good news is that there are many wholesome, delicious, and extremely nutritious foods that you may eat. Here are some of the many foods that you may enjoy on a gluten-free diet.

- Baking powder
- Baking soda
- Beans and legumes
- Corn, including corn flour, corn-meal, cornstarch
- Dairy products, including milk, cheese, and yogurt
- Eggs (fresh)
- Fish and seafood (fresh)
- Fruits and vegetables (fresh)
- Gluten-free baked goods
- Gluten-free grains, including amaranth, buckwheat, millet, quinoa, rice, sorghum, and teff
- Gluten-free pastas
- Gluten-free starches, including arrowroot, flaxseed, potato, sago, soy, and tapioca
- Gluten-free thickeners, including guar gum, lecithin, xanthan gum, and whey
- Herbs and spices
- Hominy
- Meat and poultry (fresh)
- Nuts and seeds, including nut and seed flours and butters
- Pure, natural flavorings

Foods to Avoid

Eating gluten-free means avoiding all foods that contain gluten, such as wheat, barley, and rye. The list of foods that may contain these ingredients is long and contains many foods you might never suspect. Here some foods to avoid while following the gluten-free diet.

- Beer, ale, lager
- Bran
- Breaded vegetables, seafood, and meat
- Breading, bread stuffing, bread crumbs
- Breads and baked goods made with flours that contain gluten
- Brewer's yeast
- Canned sauces and gravy mixes
- Cereal, granola bars, and breakfast pastries
- Couscous
- Crackers, pretzels, cookies, and other snack foods that are not certified gluten-free
- Flavored coffees and teas
- Grains and flours that contain gluten, including atta, barley, bulgur, dinkel, durum, kamut, einkorn, emmer, farina, farro, graham, rye, semolina, spelt, triticale, and wheat
- Hydrolyzed wheat protein
- Imitation bacon bits
- Malt, malt extract, malt syrup, malt flavoring, malt vinegar, and malted milk
- Matzo, matzo meal
- Modified wheat starch
- Orzo
- Panko
- Pastas that are not certified gluten-free
- Processed foods
- Seitan and fu (common meat substitutes that are made from wheat gluten)
- Udon

Ten Tips to Make Going Gluten-Free Easier

1. **Focus on what you *can* eat, not on what you can't.** Rather than getting down about how miserable your life is going to be without pasta, bread, cakes, and cookies, embrace all those foods you can still eat (rice, quinoa, potatoes, cheese, fresh fruit, and so on). Have fun discovering gluten-free substitutes.
2. **Learn to love your kitchen.** Yes, you can eat out and still eat gluten-free, but it isn't easy. Learning to cook a few fantastic gluten-free dishes and mastering the use of a handful of gluten-free alternative ingredients will transform your meals from dreary exercises in deprivation into fun adventures of discovery.
3. **Get used to planning ahead.** Make lists, do your grocery shopping, plan your meals in advance, pack lunches to take with you to work or school, and make sure you always have gluten-free snacks on hand.

4. **Enjoy healthy fats.** Fat gives you a feeling of fullness and satisfaction, so don't skimp on it when you are transitioning to a gluten-free diet. Just make sure to choose healthy monounsaturated fats that are full of omega-3 fatty acids. Good sources of healthy fat include avocadoes and avocado oil; coconut, coconut milk, coconut cream, coconut oil, and coconut butter; nuts and seeds (almonds, walnuts, hazelnuts, cashews, pumpkin seeds, and so on); and nut and seed butters.

5. **Embrace a wide variety of fresh foods.** Don't jump into the gluten-free life by stocking up on gluten-free bread, crackers, and cookies and continuing to eat just as you always have, minus the gluten. For one thing, gluten-free substitutes are often loaded with fat and sugar (to make up for the flavor lost when the wheat is cut out). They are also expensive and often less nutritious than their whole-grain counterparts. Instead, ease into the gluten-free lifestyle by loading up on the wide variety of fresh, healthy foods that are still available to you. Visit your local farmers' market and stock up on fresh fruits and vegetables. Buy fresh meat, chicken, eggs, dairy, and fish, which are naturally gluten-free.

6. **Get to know your neighborhood natural foods store.** Natural foods stores carry lots of gluten-free foods, including gluten-free breads and other baked goods. So do many supermarkets. Some grocery stores will provide you with a list of the gluten-free products they carry, so be sure to ask.

7. **Discover new cuisines.** Italian (pasta, pizza) and Chinese (soy sauce) are challenging for the gluten-free foodie, but there are plenty of delicious cuisines that use very few ingredients with gluten in their cooking. Indian, Thai, and Vietnamese, especially, have lots of gluten-free options.

8. **Substitute whole foods for pasta and bread.** Keep in mind that many gluten-free substitutes contain a lot of empty calories. Whole foods such as brown rice, potatoes, polenta, and quinoa make nutritious side dishes and taste great.

9. **Stay up-to-date on the latest gluten-free news.** There are numerous magazines that focus on gluten-free living, including *Living Without, Simply Gluten Free,* and *Delight,* to name just a few. And don't forget the blogosphere. *Gluten-Free Girl, Gluten-Free Goddess, Elana's Pantry, Gluten-Free Mommy, Celiac Chicks, Book of Yum,* and *No Gluten, No Problem* are just a few of the great blogs that offer gluten-free recipes, product reviews, and tips for living a gluten-free life.

10. **Create a supportive community.** Having someone to compare notes with can make the gluten-free journey a whole lot more fun. If you have friends who are gluten-free, ask them to join you in exploring cooking techniques, products, and restaurants. If you don't know a soul who has given up gluten, go online. There are forums where you can chat with others who are gluten-free, as well as meetups in many areas where you might make a real-life friend or two to join you on the journey.

SNEAKY GLUTEN PRODUCTS

Maintaining a strict gluten-free diet requires constant vigilance. Gluten can (and does) pop up in surprising places. For instance, many ingredients in processed foods—fillers, thickeners, and emulsifiers—contain gluten.

Fortunately, federal food labeling laws require that any product that contains wheat or wheat-based ingredients must list them on the label. With diligent attention to ingredient lists, you can avoid wheat-based products. Unfortunately, the same is not true for products made with rye or barley, which also contain gluten. If you are serious about avoiding gluten, watch out for the products listed below.

Not all versions of these products contain gluten, but some do. Read the labels carefully, and if you're still not sure, contact the manufacturer. Or look for versions of these products that are labeled as gluten-free.

- Aged cheeses, including blue cheese
- Alcoholic beverages, flavored
- Artificial flavors and colors
- Art supplies, such as paints, Play-Doh, and clay
- Baked beans, canned
- Bottled salad dressings, which may contain malt vinegar and/or thickeners
- Bottled sauces, such as Worcestershire
- Bouillon cubes
- Broths, canned and concentrated
- Chewing gum
- Chocolate, licorice, and other candies
- Cleaning products, especially dish soap, dishwasher detergent, "soft" cleansers, and bar soaps
- Coffee and tea that contain artificial flavors

- Cosmetics, including many lipsticks
- Dried fruits, if they are processed using machines that also process ingredients with gluten
- French fries, if the oil they're fried in is contaminated by battered ingredients such as onions rings or chicken nuggets
- Glues and adhesives, including postage stamps, stickers, and envelopes
- Ice cream, including obvious flavors with gluten-containing ingredients, such as cookies and brownies, as well as the less obvious varieties that contain wheat-derived thickeners
- Imitation crab meat (aka surimi)
- Instant coffee
- Ketchup
- Licorice and other candies
- Modified food starch

- Mustard; the bright yellow kind you find at ballparks across the country almost always contains wheat flour
- Nuts, if they are processed using machines that also process ingredients with gluten
- Oats, oatmeal, oat bran, oat flour—unless they are specified as pure, uncontaminated oats, which don't contain gluten; oats are often milled on equipment that also processes wheat, leading to cross-contamination
- Pickles; some are seasoned with gluten-containing vinegars, such as malt vinegar
- Pills and capsules
- Potato chips, flavored
- Processed meats, including lunch meats, hot dogs, sausages, meatballs, and bacon
- Rotisserie chicken and self-basting poultry
- Seasoning mixes and spice blends, such as curry powder, and dried seasonings, such as mustard powder
- Soy sauce and tamari, which are often fermented with wheat
- Toiletries, including shampoos, conditioners, lotions, facial cleansers, sun protection products, toothpaste, and mouthwash
- Tomato sauce and paste
- Vinegar, nondistilled
- Vitamins and herbal supplements, which often include fillers such as modified food starch
- Wasabi paste, which often includes gluten-containing thickeners
- Yeast, which may be grown on a wheat-based substrate
- Yogurts, flavored

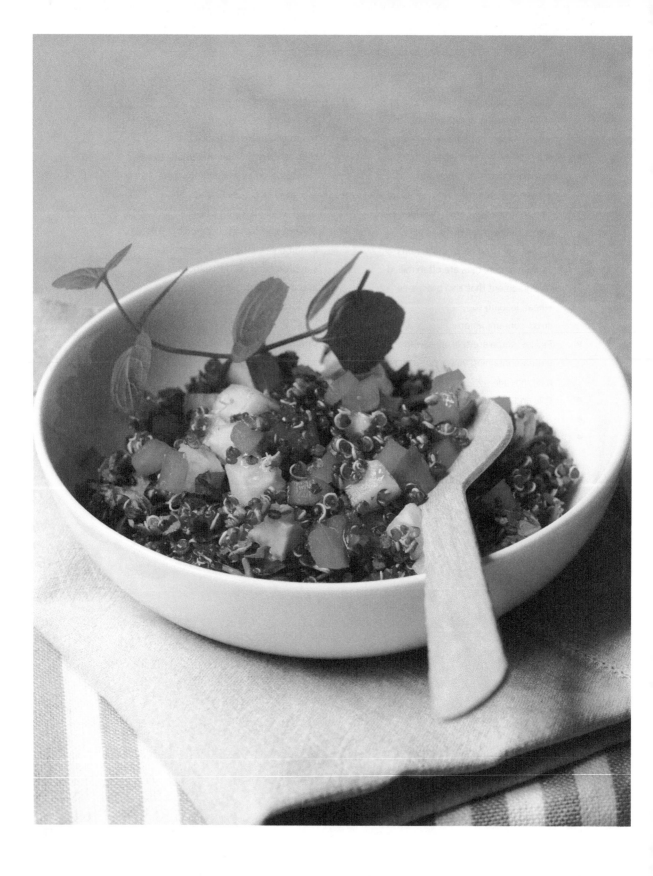

2

Quick and Easy Gluten-Free Cooking

By now you understand the basics of the gluten-free diet, including which foods you may enjoy and which to avoid. Now it's time to transfer these guidelines into real life. You need to get dinner on the table—and lunch and breakfast, too. This chapter will help you figure out how to do so, without spending hours in the kitchen or breaking the bank.

There are many sources of information—books, blogs, websites, and more—about gluten-free living. Unfortunately, some of these resources assume that you have all the time in the world to research foods, find alternatives and substitutes for gluten products, search out hard-to-find ingredients and then pay through the nose for them, and labor over complicated recipes. But it doesn't have to be that way. Adopting a gluten-free lifestyle does not require you to give up your day job or drain your savings account.

This chapter provides tips and advice for making gluten-free meals quickly and easily. Here you'll find information on the handful of specialty ingredients that will prove good investments and advice on shopping for affordable gluten-free ingredients, planning your meals, cooking, and stocking your pantry so that a delicious gluten-free meal is always just minutes away.

Plan Ahead

As with any diet, meal plan, or lifestyle change, the biggest key to success is planning ahead. You'll need to stock up on certain gluten-free foods and change up your day-to-day meal plan.

Start by planning the meals you'll eat for the next week. Look through the recipes in part 2 of this book, as well as other sources, and decide what you'll eat each day for breakfast, lunch, and dinner. Don't forget to think about snacks—both substantial snacks to serve as mini-meals as well as those little nibbles that tide you over between meals.

While it may seem tedious to write out a one-week meal plan, it will ultimately save you time, not to mention money, when you know exactly what you are going to eat and can make a shopping list to ensure you get everything you need in one shopping trip. Having a meal plan can also help you make the most of leftovers, adding to the time- and money-saving benefits.

Many of your meals can be put together out of simple ingredients. You can also cook more than you need for one meal and eat the leftovers for several meals. For example, roast a chicken one night and serve it with roasted or steamed vegetables. The next day's breakfast can be scrambled eggs with leftover veggies. For lunch, have a salad with leftover chicken.

Make a Shopping List

When you have your meal plan ready to go, make a detailed shopping list. Be sure to include every ingredient for every dish or snack you plan to prepare. Then check your pantry to see what you already have and cross those items off the list.

You'll obviously want to shop every week for fresh proteins (meat, fish, dairy), vegetables, fruits, nuts, and seeds.

As for specialty ingredients, many gluten-free cookbooks call for flour substitutes that may or may not be available at your local markets. The recipes here mostly use everyday ingredients that are sure to be available at your supermarket: meats, vegetables, fruits, nuts, and so on. When specialty flours are called for, we've kept it to the most commonly available choices, like rice flour and almond meal. You can also use the recipe for Homemade Gluten-Free All-Purpose Flour Blend (page 32) or the other gluten-free flours (recipes start on page 29) to make your own mix that can be used in a wide array of recipes.

Gluten-Free Pantry Staples

A well-stocked pantry makes the transition to gluten-free cooking as easy as possible. By having certain gluten-free staples on hand, you'll be able to create delicious meals that satisfy both your dietary limitations and your desire for great-tasting food. In addition to all the elements of a normal well-stocked pantry (quality cooking and salad oils, vinegars, spices, herbs, and so on), the following items will ensure that you can make satisfying gluten-free meals at home.

All oils are not created equal. Olive oil, which is full of healthy monounsaturated fats, is great for salad dressings and other uncooked dishes, but it burns when heated to high temperatures. Coconut oil is also loaded with healthy fats, but it doesn't burn at high temperatures, so it's great for cooking. Look for unrefined, virgin, organic, cold-pressed coconut oil for the best quality. This can be found at natural foods stores, and most supermarkets now carry it, as well.

Bread and Wrap Replacements

When you get rid of gluten, you are left with a sandwich dilemma: How do you make a portable, handheld lunch without bread? Luckily, there are plenty of gluten-free bread alternatives as well as gluten-free breads.

- Gluten-free corn tortillas are not just for tacos. They make the perfect holder for just about any sandwich or wrap fillings. Brown rice tortillas are more similar to flour tortillas, making them a perfect substitute wrap for burritos. You can also cut them up and toast them to make crispy, crunchy chips for dipping or crackers for topping.
- Nori sheets and rice wrappers can be used to make your own gluten-free sushi, spring rolls, and egg rolls. Large lettuce or cabbage leaves are great holders for saucier foods and add a bit of crunch.

Gluten-Free Broth

Many store-bought broths contain gluten in the form of natural flavorings or other additives, so either make your own or read the label carefully before buying. Stock up on gluten-free chicken, beef, or vegetable broth in cans or cartons, broth concentrate, or bouillon cubes. They are great for quickly adding depth of flavor to many dishes.

Gluten-Free Flours and Meals

Wheat is not the only flour that can be used for baking, thickening sauces, or breading meat, fish, and veggies. Gluten-free flours are often used in blends to get the best of each. Try out different flours and decide which you like best.

- Grain-based flours include rice (white, brown, sweet), millet, teff, sorghum, quinoa, amaranth, and others. They tend to be high in fiber and low in fat. They work well as substitutes in baked goods and can be used to thicken sauces and dredge meats and vegetables before browning.

- Nut and seed flours—including almond or hazelnut—add extra protein and healthy fats. They're great for baked goods when you want a hearty, moist texture. Coconut flour is full of fiber and healthy fats and can be used in combination with other alternative flours to replace the wheat flour in cookies, muffins, and breads.
- Bean flours—chickpea, lentil, fava—are often used in Middle Eastern and Indian cooking and can be used to replace some of the grain-based flour in baking recipes to add extra protein and fiber.
- Gluten-free all-purpose flour is a combination of gluten-free flours that you can use to whip up pancakes, muffins, cookies, or cakes at a moment's notice. You can also use it to bread chicken or fish before panfrying. There are numerous brands of gluten-free all-purpose flour on the market, or you can make your own (see the recipe on page 32).

Gluten-Free Pasta and Crackers

There are many varieties on the market these days, including pastas made from rice, corn, quinoa, and other grains. Try them all and decide which you like best.

- Gluten-free crackers are nice to have around when you need a quick snack or something to add to a cheese plate when guests drop by.

Gluten-Free Sauces and Condiments

As mentioned in chapter 1, many sauces and condiments are thickened or flavored with products made from wheat. Read labels carefully and look for gluten-free alternatives, then stock up.

- Get some gluten-free tamari or soy sauce to zip up recipes and for dipping. Make sure you check the label because many tamari sauces contain wheat. Or you can try coconut aminos—a slightly salty condiment that's made from coconut tree sap. You'll find it to be a fantastic gluten-free alternative to soy sauce. Look for it in health food stores and online.
- Stock up on some good gluten-free seasoning mixes, as well, for when you don't feel like doing anything more than shaking some spices from the package into the pot.

Gluten-Free Thickeners

Thickeners are used to mimic the function of gluten in many gluten-free baking recipes, and they can also be used in place of flour to thicken sauces and soups. Arrowroot and cornstarch are often used to thicken sauces. Tapioca and potato starch are also common thickeners in gluten-free baking recipes. These are relatively easy to find in the supermarket.

- Xanthan gum or guar gum help to bind, stabilize, emulsify, thicken, and lend structure to gluten-free baked goods. You can buy these products in powdered form at natural foods or health food stores.
- Psyllium husk is a natural fiber that works in a similar way to xanthan and guar gums. Some people who are sensitive to gluten are also sensitive to gums, and for them, psyllium husk is a great alternative.

Nuts and Seeds

These can be added to salads instead of croutons or eaten as a snack instead of pretzels or other foods with gluten.

- Almonds and hazelnuts can be ground into a flour for baking. Cashews can also be blended in a food processor or blender with a bit of water and used as a great gluten-free thickener for soups, sauces, and stews.

Potatoes

Simple spuds can replace pasta or bread in many meals. Try branching out from the good old russet or Idaho potato. Baby red potatoes, fingerlings, Peruvian purples, and others offer great variety.

Gluten-Free Whole Grains

While wheat-based pasta and cereals are off the menu, there is a whole other world of grains available in your supermarket. These offer flavor, variety, and, in many cases, far more nutrition than wheat.

- Rice is a great substitute for pasta and offers nearly as much variety: brown, basmati, jasmine, arborio, red, black, and sticky rice all have different flavors and textures to round out meals of various cuisines.
- Quinoa is the only grain that has a complete protein, and it works well as a hot side dish substitute for pasta or couscous, cold in salads, or even cooked and lightly sweetened with fruit or maple syrup for a satisfying hot breakfast cereal.
- Other grains, such as millet, amaranth, buckwheat (despite its name, this grain really is gluten-free), corn, and oats (make sure to buy gluten-free oats), can make great side dishes and hot cereals.

GLUTEN-FREE ALTERNATIVES

You don't have to shell out lots of money for store-bought gluten-free versions of your old standbys. In many cases, there's a supermarket staple that can be swapped for the version that contains gluten. For other foods, you can whip up your own homemade version.

Bread, Rolls, and Buns

Corn tortillas (make sure you're using a gluten-free version), lettuce leaves, or blanched kale or collard greens make great substitutes for wrapping up sandwich ingredients, including hot dogs and burgers.

Bread Crumbs

Whirl gluten-free oats in a food processor or crush gluten-free cereal flakes for bread crumbs. Season them as you wish and use them to coat meat, fish, or vegetables before panfrying or baking to a crispy golden brown.

Couscous

Remember, couscous is a wheat-based pasta, not a grain. Quinoa, shredded and steamed cauliflower, or polenta can all be substituted successfully.

Pasta

There are lots of gluten-free pasta brands on the market made from rice, corn, quinoa, and other grains. Vegetables such as spaghetti squash, zucchini, parsnips, and butternut squash also make delicious, low-carb pasta alternatives when cut into thin ribbons.

Pizza Crust

If you can't live without pizza, try making a crust of mashed potatoes mixed with a bit of gluten-free flour, spread thin and toasted in a hot oven until crispy. Cauliflower chopped fine in a food processor, steamed, and mixed with a bit of gluten-free flour and cheese works well, too, and is also low-carb.

Tortilla Chips or Crackers

Toasted brown rice or corn tortillas work well as either crackers (try them topped with cheese) or tortilla chips (dip them in guacamole, salsa, hummus, or veggie dips).

GLUTEN-FREE FLOUR CONVERSIONS

These days, the array of wheat-free flours available at most supermarkets is mind-boggling. Grain-based wheat-free flours such as amaranth, buckwheat, brown rice, and sorghum take some getting used to when baking with them, but with a good recipe, they turn out surprisingly good breads, cakes, and other baked goods. Coconut flour is high in fiber and won't cause your blood sugar to spike, but it's very dry, so a little goes a long way in a recipe. Low-carb nut-based flours like almond and hazelnut deliver good doses of protein and omega-3 fatty acids, and they add a rich, nutty flavor, too.

What if you want to convert one of your old flour-based recipes to one that is gluten-free? It absolutely can be done. Some recipes are easier to convert than others, but with a bit of trial and error, you can successfully make most recipes gluten-free. Here is a simple conversion formula.

- **Replace 1 cup of wheat flour with ½ cup of gluten-free flour of your choice (this can be a combination of flours) plus ½ cup of starch (most commonly, a 50-50 combination of potato starch and tapioca starch).** For example: 1 cup wheat flour = ¼ cup sorghum flour + ¼ cup brown rice flour + ¼ cup potato starch + ¼ cup tapioca starch.

Use the following table for other gluten-free flour conversion ratios.

Helpful Tools and Equipment

If you like to cook, you probably already have all the tools you need for gluten-free cooking. But if you are setting up your kitchen for the first time or are looking to beef up your kitchen equipment—perhaps expecting to be doing more cooking at home—here are a few items many gluten-free cooks find useful.

Essential

- **Dutch oven.** A Dutch oven is a heavy cooking pot with a lid. They are the workhorses of the kitchen. Appropriate for both the stove top and a hot oven, they are indispensable for cooking up pots of risotto, quinoa, and beans or for braising meats and even making roasts.

GLUTEN-FREE FLOUR	EQUIVALENT TO 1 CUP WHEAT FLOUR	PROPERTIES	BEST USE	HOW TO STORE
Almond flour	½ cup	Sweet, nutty flavor; high in protein; rough texture	Cakes, cookies, and cupcakes where a nutty flavor and rough texture is desired	Tightly sealed in the freezer
Amaranth flour	⅞ cup	Earthy, nutty flavor; high in calcium, protein, iron, and fiber	Savory breads and baked goods like pizza dough or crust for quiches or savory tarts	Tightly sealed in the refrigerator or freezer
Brown rice flour	⅞ cup	Moderately strong, slightly nutty flavor; high in fiber; fairly grainy	Most baked goods, especially cookies and other delicate baked goods; use in combination with other flours to avoid gumminess (use 50 percent rice flour)	Tightly sealed in the refrigerator
Buckwheat flour	1 cup	Strong flavor	Breads and rolls; use in combination with other flours (use 50 percent buckwheat flour to impart a hearty whole-wheat-like flavor to breads)	Tightly sealed in the refrigerator
Coconut flour	1 cup	High in fiber; low in carbohydrates; very dry, strong flavor	Cakes and cupcakes to create low-carb versions; leavening with eggs is essential; add one extra egg to the recipe for each ¼ cup of coconut flour used; add in small quantities to other flours to increase fiber and decrease carb content	Tightly sealed in the freezer
Millet flour	¾ cup	Moderately strong, sweet, and slightly nutty flavor; high in protein and fiber; fine grain	Light baked goods such as yeast breads, pizza crusts, and flatbread; use in combination with other flours (no more than 25 percent millet flour)	Tightly sealed in the refrigerator or freezer
Quinoa flour	1 cup	Delicate, nutty flavor; high in protein; moderately grainy	Cookies, cakes, and breads to increase nutritional content; use in combination with other flours (use up to 25 percent quinoa flour)	Tightly sealed in the refrigerator
Sorghum flour	1 cup	Moderately mild, slightly sweet flavor; high in protein; minimally grainy	Pancakes, breads, muffins, and cookies, especially where a darker appearance is desired, such as in brown breads or gingersnaps; use in combination with other flours (use 25 to 30 percent sorghum flour)	Tightly sealed at room temperature or in the refrigerator
Teff flour	⅞ cup	Mild, slightly nutty flavor; high in fiber, protein, and calcium; fine grain	Pancakes, waffles, quick breads, cookies, and cakes	Tightly sealed in the refrigerator
White rice flour	⅞ cup	Very mild flavor; very grainy	Most baked goods, especially cookies and other delicate baked goods; best used in combination with other flours to avoid gumminess (use 50 percent rice flour)	Tightly sealed in the refrigerator

- **Fine-mesh colander.** You may already have one with larger holes for draining pasta, but the fine mesh is important for rinsing small grains like millet and quinoa.
- **Good knives.** Purchase a cleaver, a paring knife, and a large serrated knife for cutting loaves of bread. They should feel comfortable and well balanced in your hand. Then get a little handheld knife sharpener, and keep your knives sharp; knives are easier and safer to use when well honed.
- **Large cutting board.** No slicing and dicing on a plate; it will ruin your knives and your plate. Wood or plastic is up to you. You should consider investing in cutting boards for meats and non-meat options as bacteria from meat can contaminate vegetables.
- **Loaf pan.** If you want to make your own gluten-free sandwich bread, a standard-size loaf pan is a necessary tool. It works well for meatloaf and other dishes, as well.
- **Nonstick baking sheets.** You may end up doing a lot more baking than you're used to, since gluten-free versions of your favorites may be hard to come by or expensive. A couple of good nonstick full or half baking sheets will see a lot of use.
- **Skillet.** Purchase a good, heavy 10-inch skillet. You'll use it for everything from omelets to stir-fries. Consider getting a nonstick skillet for the stove top and a cast-iron one for foods you want to sear at high heat (meat, for example) and dishes that go from stove top to oven.

Important

- **Digital scale.** A good digital scale is handy for converting standard baking recipes to gluten-free. Gluten-free flours vary widely in terms of weight, so substituting them cup for cup (by volume) for regular wheat flour can be risky. Using a good digital scale and substituting by weight (gram for gram) is a much safer bet.
- **Food processor.** High-quality food processors are expensive, but they'll save you hours of chopping and mincing time in the kitchen. They can also be used to make your own gluten-free flours, meals, and nut butters.
- **High-powered blender.** These are great for making your own nut meals and flours, and they also turn out fantastic smoothies.
- **Instant-read digital thermometer.** These come in handy when determining when meat is done, and they work well for baked goods, too.

Nice to Have

- **Bread machine.** It may seem contradictory that you'll be baking more bread now that you are eating gluten-free, but if you want to make your own gluten-free breads (which will save you money and give you control over the ingredients), a bread machine is a huge time-saver. You can often find lightly used bread machines at thrift stores or garage sales.

- **Pasta maker.** Like bread machines, pasta makers give you the power to make your own gluten-free noodles exactly to your liking. Also like bread machines, they are often easy to find for an attractive price at garage sales and thrift stores.

- **Rice cooker.** A rice cooker can be used to cook rice, obviously, but it also works well for quinoa and other grains. Best of all, you can set it and forget it while you cook the rest of the meal.

- **Slow cooker.** The ultimate set-it-and-forget-it kitchen tool, the slow cooker enables you to combine ingredients in the morning, push a button, and let the machine cook your dinner while you're at work. This will save you time and make gluten-free dinners less of a chore.

- **Spring-loaded ice cream scoop.** These are useful for scooping muffin batter into tins or scooping uniform-size cookie dough balls or biscuits onto baking sheets.

- **Stand mixer.** This is another big-ticket item, but one that you'll wonder how you ever lived without. This handy machine blends thoroughly—which is especially important when baking without gluten—and frees up your hands to do other work while the dough is being blended.

Tips for Gluten-Free Cooking and Baking

Gluten-free cooking isn't all that different from regular cooking, but it may take some time and practice to get used to using gluten-free alternatives, like wheat-free flours and starches. Here's a list of cooking and baking tips to help you get started on the gluten-free diet.

- **For the best results, use recipes that are meant to be gluten-free.** Many recipes can be converted, but some that were developed to use wheat flour, for instance, won't translate well.

- **Use puréed fruits or vegetables.** Puréed fruits and vegetables—applesauce, bananas, even black beans or beets—add moisture, flavor, and structure (thanks to pectin, a natural thickener found in the cell walls of plants). Try replacing part of the liquid or fat in a recipe with fruit or veggies, and you'll also boost the nutrition a bit.

- **Boost flavorings.** Increase the amount of vanilla or other extract or spices to make up for some of the flavor lost along with the wheat. Start small, adding just a touch more the first time. You can always increase the amount the next time, if you want an even bigger boost.

- **Make large batches of breads, pizza crusts, and other baked goods.** Dough can be frozen and then thawed and cooked as needed. Pizza crusts and flatbreads can be partly baked and then topped and baked whenever you need a quick meal. Freeze raw cookie dough in balls on a baking sheet and then transfer them to a freezer-safe zipper plastic bag. When a craving strikes, bake as few or as many cookies as you like. Other baked goods, such as rolls, cakes, and sweet breads, freeze well after baking.

- **Chop once, cook all week.** When chopping vegetables such as onions, celery, and peppers for cooking, chop more than you need and store the extra in zipper plastic bags to use in other meals throughout the week.

- **Save scraps for stock.** Save all those ugly bits—onion cores, carrot ends, etc.— as well as chicken bones and even Parmesan cheese rinds in small zipper plastic bags in the freezer and use them for making homemade stock. When you want to whip up a quick soup or sauce, you're already ahead of the game.

- **Freeze extra ginger and garlic.** Freezing makes both ginger and garlic last longer, and they're easier to grate when frozen, too. Peel first and then store extra ginger and garlic in zipper plastic bags.

- **Go for a nice brown crust.** Dredge meats and vegetables in almond flour or coconut flour before cooking to create a nicely browned crust and to naturally thicken soups and stews with meat in them.

- **Experiment with bread crumb substitutes.** Try using boxed mashed potato mix, gluten-free oats (whirled in a food processor), or crushed gluten-free cereal as an alternative to bread crumbs in your favorite recipes.

- **Buy gluten-free flours in large bags and store them in the refrigerator or freezer.** You'll save money and always have what you need on hand.

- **Use gluten-free flours in combination.** When attempting to recreate a wheat-based favorite, mixing up flours is essential. This is because no gluten-free flour on its own can perfectly imitate the flavor and texture of wheat flour. By combining two or more flours, you can get the best qualities of each, bringing you closer to the flavor and texture of the original.

- **Make a big batch of Homemade Gluten-Free All-Purpose Flour Blend** (page 32). Use this blend anywhere gluten-free all-purpose flour is called for. With a little tweaking and the addition of ingredients like xanthan gum or psyllium husk powder, this blend can be used to replace all-purpose flour in many standard recipes, as well.

- **Turn your Homemade Gluten-Free All-Purpose Flour Blend into self-rising flour.** Just add 1½ teaspoons of baking powder and ½ teaspoon of sea salt to each cup of gluten-free flour mix.

- **Create your own test kitchen.** Bake up a small portion of the recipe, like one muffin, to see how it turns out. You can make adjustments to the rest of the batter, if needed, before baking the rest.

- **Forget separating wet and dry ingredients.** To get a moist crumb when baking with gluten-free flours, forget the old rule about creaming the fat and sugar together first, before adding the dry ingredients. Instead, put everything—sugar, flours, starch, eggs, flavorings—in the bowl at the same time and mix.

- **Don't skimp on fat.** Gluten-free flours are often drier than wheat flour and the end result can be crumblier. Adding more fat—butter, coconut oil, vegetable oil—adds moisture and holds it all together.

- **Xanthan gum (or guar gum) is a key ingredient in gluten-free baking.** It simulates the binding action of gluten in wheat-based baked goods. Gluten holds everything together in standard baked goods. When you leave it out, you need to replace it with something to keep your baked goods from being too crumbly. Remember, a little gum goes a long way and too much could make the end result, well, gummy. Check the ingredients label of gluten-free baking mixes because many already include xanthan gum.

- **Lighten up.** Gluten-free flours often produce a denser product than wheat flour. To counter this, try increasing the leavening agents. Add a touch more baking powder, baking soda, or yeast; add an extra egg or two; replace some of the liquid with yogurt or buttermilk; or try using carbonated water in place of some or all of the liquid.

- **Make sure your baking powder is gluten-free.** Not all of them are. If you can't find a gluten-free version, you can make your own by combining equal parts baking soda and cream of tartar.

TROUBLE-SHOOTING YOUR GLUTEN-FREE BAKING

Gluten-free baking can be tricky. If you've been baking with wheat all your life, it takes some adjustment in your thinking to convert to gluten-free baking. Here are a few common problems gluten-free bakers run up against and how to fix them.

- **Your baked goods are too crumbly or lack structure.**
  When you leave out the gluten, you have to replace it with something that will provide similar stretching and binding characteristics. Xanthan gum is an emulsifier that does just that. You'll find xanthan gum in the baking aisle of any natural foods store. It's pricey, but a little goes a long way; most recipes call for between ¼ and ¾ teaspoon per cup of flour.

- **Your goodies are too grainy.**
  Some gluten-free flours (we're looking at you, rice flour) are especially grainy, while others are more delicate (ah, teff, our powdery friend). When baking delicate baked goods such as cupcakes, use a gluten-free flour or flour blend that is on the less grainy end of the spectrum. The popular gluten-free flours, listed from least grainy to grainiest: almond, coconut, buckwheat, teff, millet, sorghum, amaranth, quinoa, brown rice, white rice.

- **Your baked goods are too dry.**
  Many gluten-free flours contain less moisture than wheat flour, so to keep your results from turning out overly dry, add additional moisture, such as an extra egg or a bit more fat, or replace white sugar with a more moist sweetener, such as rice syrup, agave, honey, or brown sugar. Or add a little applesauce or other puréed fruit.

- **The flavor is too bland.** Many gluten-free flours, such as white rice and teff flour, are less flavorful than wheat or rye flour. To boost the flavor of savory baked goods, choose a flour with more intense flavor, such as quinoa or amaranth. For sweets, bumping up the quantity of spices, extracts, or other flavorings can make a big difference.

- **Your yeast breads, quick breads, or cakes are too dense.** Gluten-free flours generally need more leavening than wheat flour. For a lighter result, you can increase the amount of baking soda, baking powder, or yeast in your recipe, or try adding other ingredients that function as leaven, such as buttermilk or even club soda.

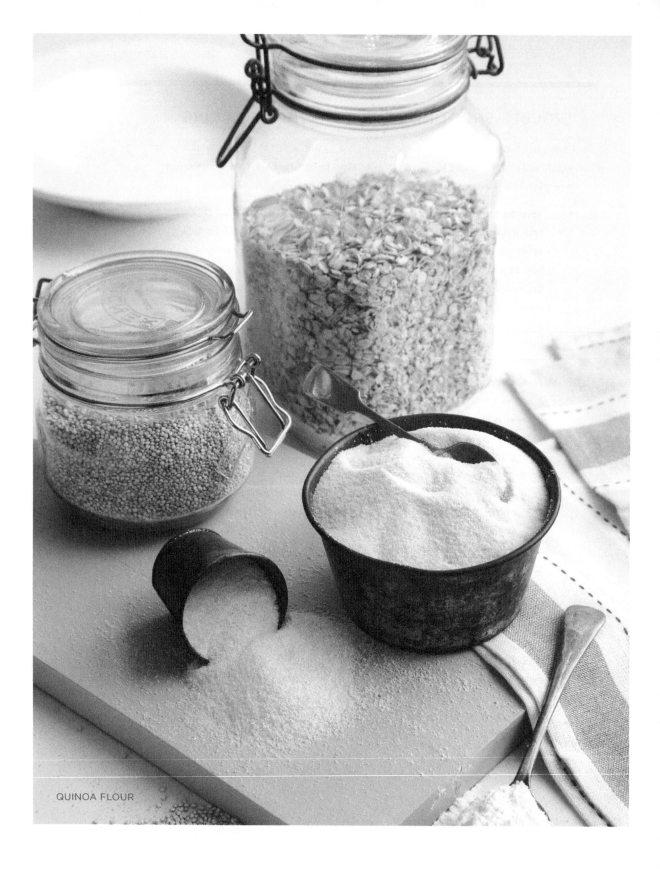

QUINOA FLOUR

3

Homemade Gluten-Free Flours

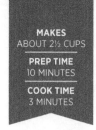

MAKES
ABOUT 2½ CUPS

PREP TIME
10 MINUTES

COOK TIME
3 MINUTES

Homemade Quinoa Flour

Quinoa flour is one of the most nutritious flours you can get, offering complete protein as well as fiber and many other nutrients. Use it to replace some of the other flour in your recipes for cookies, cakes, or breads to add a nutritional boost. Quinoa flour can be substituted in a one-to-one ratio for all-purpose flour, but don't use more than about 25 percent quinoa flour in a recipe or the taste could be overpowering.

Cooking tip The best tool for making grain flours is a grain mill, which is made just for that job. But a spice grinder, food processor, or high-powered blender will work, as well.

3 CUPS DRIED QUINOA

1. Toast the dry quinoa in a large skillet over medium heat, stirring occasionally, until it begins to make a slight popping sound and smells toasty, about 3 minutes.

2. Transfer the quinoa to the grinder or food processor and process it on high speed until it becomes a fine powder.

3. Store the flour in a tightly sealed container in the refrigerator or freezer.

NUTRITIONAL INFORMATION PER ½ CUP: CALORIES 295   TOTAL FAT 4.8G   SATURATED FAT 0.6G
TRANS FAT 0.0G   SODIUM 4MG   TOTAL CARBOHYDRATES 51.3G   SUGARS 0.0G   PROTEIN 11.3G

Homemade Almond Flour

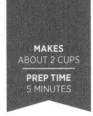

MAKES
ABOUT 2 CUPS

PREP TIME
5 MINUTES

Almond flour is full of protein and heart-healthy omega-3 fatty acids. But store-bought almond flour is pricey, and it can go rancid quickly. It's easy to make at home using blanched almonds and a food processor or high-powered blender. Be careful, though, because in just seconds, your beautiful almond flour can turn into almond butter.

3 CUPS BLANCHED, UNSALTED ALMONDS

1. Place the almonds in the food processor or blender and pulse them to a fine flour.

2. Store the flour in a tightly sealed container in the refrigerator.

NUTRITIONAL INFORMATION PER ½ CUP: CALORIES 412 TOTAL FAT 35.6G SATURATED FAT 2.7G
TRANS FAT 0.0G SODIUM 1MG TOTAL CARBOHYDRATES 15.3G SUGARS 0.0G PROTEIN 15.1G

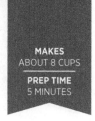
Homemade Gluten-Free All-Purpose Flour Blend

Mix up a large batch of this flour blend, and you'll be able to whip up all sorts of baked goods quickly and easily. This is a versatile mix that works well for a lot of different recipes. Feel free to experiment to find your own perfect blend. You can use this mix for any recipe in this book that calls for gluten-free all-purpose flour.

Ingredient tip Want to be able to whip up a batch of pancakes, waffles, or biscuits in a flash on Sunday morning? Adding 1½ teaspoons of baking powder and ½ teaspoon of salt to each cup of Gluten-Free All-Purpose Flour Blend turns it into a self-rising baking mix, similar to the pancake and waffle mixes you buy at the supermarket.

4¾ CUPS PLUS ⅓ CUP WHITE
    RICE FLOUR

1⅔ CUPS BROWN RICE FLOUR

1⅓ CUPS POTATO STARCH

¾ CUP TAPIOCA STARCH

1. Whisk together the white rice flour, brown rice flour, potato starch, and tapioca starch.

2. Store the flour in an airtight container in the refrigerator.

NUTRITIONAL INFORMATION PER ½ CUP: CALORIES 335 TOTAL FAT 1.2G SATURATED FAT 0.0G
TRANS FAT 0.0G SODIUM 3MG TOTAL CARBOHYDRATES 75.0G SUGARS 0.0G PROTEIN 4.1G

NOTES

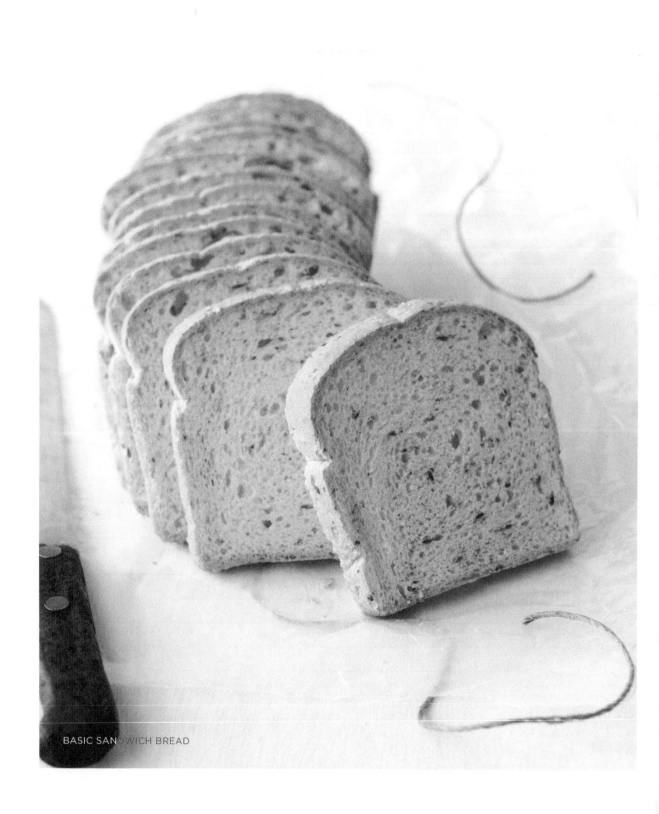

BASIC SANDWICH BREAD

4

Breads and Sandwiches

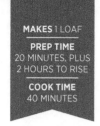
Basic Sandwich Bread

If you thought going gluten-free would mean saying good-bye to all your favorite sandwiches, think again. This recipe delivers a classic sandwich bread that's perfect for all your old standbys.

3 CUPS GLUTEN-FREE ALL-
   PURPOSE FLOUR
3 TABLESPOONS SUGAR
2 TEASPOONS INSTANT DRY YEAST
1¼ TEASPOONS SALT
1¼ TEASPOONS XANTHAN GUM

1 CUP WARM MILK
¼ CUP UNSALTED BUTTER, AT ROOM
   TEMPERATURE
3 EGGS
NONSTICK COOKING SPRAY

1. In a large bowl using an electric hand mixer or in the bowl of your stand mixer, combine the flour, sugar, yeast, salt, and xanthan gum.

2. With the mixer running, add the milk in a thin stream and mix until the dough comes together. Add the butter and beat to mix well.

3. Add the eggs one at a time, mixing after each addition to thoroughly incorporate.

4. With the mixer set on high, beat the mixture for 3 minutes, until the batter is very smooth and thick.

5. Cover the bowl with a clean dish towel and let it rise in a warm spot on the kitchen counter for 1 hour.

6. Spray a loaf pan with cooking spray and scrape the dough into it, deflating the dough in the process. Flatten the top of the dough with a spatula or your hand. Use the cooking spray to oil a piece of plastic wrap, then cover the pan with it. Let the dough rise in a warm spot on your kitchen counter for about 1 hour, until the dough rises over the top of the sides of the pan.

7. Preheat the oven to 350°F. Bake the bread until the top is golden brown, about 40 minutes. Cool the bread on a wire rack before slicing.

NUTRITIONAL INFORMATION PER SLICE (12 SLICES PER LOAF): CALORIES 271 TOTAL FAT 5.4G SATURATED FAT 3.0G TRANS FAT 0.0G SODIUM 526MG TOTAL CARBOHYDRATES 50.1G SUGARS 0.0G PROTEIN 4.1G

BASIC SANDWICH BREAD RECIPE

Grilled Ham and Brie with Pears

SERVES 4

PREP TIME
5 MINUTES

COOK TIME
5 TO 8 MINUTES

Creamy brie, sweet pears, and salty ham are a delectable sandwich combination. A touch of apple jelly mixed with the mustard delivers a sweet surprise. If you have a panini press, this would be a great time to break it out, but a skillet or grill pan works well, too.

1 TABLESPOON APPLE JELLY

¼ CUP DIJON MUSTARD

8 SLICES BASIC GLUTEN-FREE
    SANDWICH BREAD

8 SLICES DELI HAM (6 OUNCES TOTAL)

4 OUNCES BRIE, CHILLED AND
    THINLY SLICED

1 LARGE RIPE, FIRM PEAR, CORED AND
    THINLY SLICED

NONSTICK COOKING SPRAY

1. In a small bowl, stir together the apple jelly and mustard. Spread this mixture over one side of 4 of the bread slices.

2. Top each of the jelly-mustard bread slices with 2 slices of ham, ¼ of the cheese, and ¼ of the pear slices. Top the pears with the remaining slices of bread.

3. Spray a skillet, grill pan, or panini press with cooking spray and heat it to medium-high.

4. Place the sandwiches in the hot skillet, pan, or panini press. If using a skillet or grill pan, cover and cook the sandwiches until the underside is nicely browned, about 3 minutes. Flip the sandwiches over and cook until the second side is nicely browned and the cheese is melted, 3 to 4 minutes more. If using a panini press, close the lid and cook until the sandwiches are browned on both sides and the cheese is melted, about 5 minutes total.

5. Slice each sandwich in half diagonally and serve immediately.

NUTRITIONAL INFORMATION PER SERVING: CALORIES 402 TOTAL FAT 18.3G SATURATED FAT 7.0G
TRANS FAT 0.0G SODIUM 1,088MG TOTAL CARBOHYDRATES 40.6G SUGARS 8.0G PROTEIN 16.1G

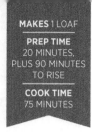

MAKES 1 LOAF

PREP TIME
20 MINUTES,
PLUS 90 MINUTES
TO RISE

COOK TIME
75 MINUTES

Seeded Multigrain Bread

This hearty bread is ideal for sandwiches packed with healthy fillings. Pile it high with egg salad, red onions, and sprouts, or use it for a gooey grilled cheese sandwich.

1 CUP PLUS 2 TABLESPOONS
    CORNSTARCH
½ CUP POTATO STARCH
½ CUP BROWN RICE FLOUR
½ CUP MILLET FLOUR
½ CUP GOLDEN FLAXSEED MEAL
¼ CUP PROTEIN POWDER
2 TABLESPOONS PSYLLIUM
    HUSK POWDER
2 TEASPOONS BAKING POWDER
1½ TEASPOONS SALT

1 TEASPOON XANTHAN GUM
2 TABLESPOONS SUGAR
1 PACKET ACTIVE DRY YEAST
½ CUP SUNFLOWER SEEDS
¼ CUP WHOLE FLAXSEEDS
3 TABLESPOONS SESAME SEEDS
2 CUPS LUKEWARM WATER
2 EGGS, AT ROOM TEMPERATURE
2 TABLESPOONS UNSALTED BUTTER,
    MELTED, PLUS MORE FOR
    PREPARING THE PAN

1. Using a mixer of your choice, whisk together the cornstarch, potato starch, rice flour, millet flour, flaxseed meal, protein powder, psyllium husk powder, baking powder, salt, xanthan gum, sugar, yeast, sunflower seeds, whole flaxseeds, and sesame seeds.

2. With the mixer set on low speed, add the water, eggs, and 2 tablespoons of butter, and beat to combine. Mix for 3 minutes with the mixer set to medium speed.

3. Grease a standard-size loaf pan with butter. Scrape the dough into the pan and flatten the top. Cover the pan with plastic wrap and let the dough rise in a warm spot in your kitchen for about 90 minutes, until the dough rises above the sides of the pan. Preheat the oven to 425°F.

4. Remove the plastic wrap from the loaf pan and bake the bread for 15 minutes.

5. Reduce the temperature to 350°F. Bake the bread for an additional 50 to 60 minutes, until the loaf is golden brown. Cool the loaf on a wire rack before slicing.

NUTRITIONAL INFORMATION PER SLICE (12 SLICES PER LOAF): CALORIES 223 TOTAL FAT 7.6G SATURATED FAT 2.0G TRANS FAT 0.0G SODIUM 611MG TOTAL CARBOHYDRATES 40.9G SUGARS 0.0G PROTEIN 6.9G

Egg Salad Sandwich with Curry, Scallions, and Watercress

SERVES 4

PREP TIME
10 MINUTES

Classic egg salad is dressed up with a dash of curry, a dollop of Dijon mustard, a sprinkling of scallions, and bits of crisp green apple. Piled on hearty Seeded Multigrain Bread, with a handful of watercress for a bit of crunch, it makes an especially satisfying lunch. Try different types of apples for a change in the flavor profile.

¼ CUP MAYONNAISE

2 TABLESPOONS SCALLIONS,
   THINLY SLICED

1 TABLESPOON MINCED SHALLOT

1½ TABLESPOONS APPLE
   CIDER VINEGAR

1½ TEASPOONS DIJON MUSTARD

¾ TEASPOON CURRY POWDER

¼ TEASPOON GROUND CUMIN

½ TEASPOON SALT

¼ TEASPOON FRESHLY GROUND
   BLACK PEPPER

4 HARDBOILED EGGS, CHOPPED

1 GRANNY SMITH APPLE, PEELED AND
   CUT INTO ⅛-INCH CUBES

8 SLICES SEEDED MULTIGRAIN BREAD

1 CUP WATERCRESS SPRIGS

1. In a medium bowl, stir together the mayonnaise, scallions, shallot, vinegar, mustard, curry powder, cumin, salt, and pepper. Add the eggs and apple and fold gently to mix.

2. Spread the egg mixture evenly on 4 slices of bread. Top each with ¼ cup of watercress and the remaining 4 bread slices.

3. Slice each sandwich in half diagonally and serve immediately.

NUTRITIONAL INFORMATION PER SERVING: CALORIES 433 TOTAL FAT 12.5G SATURATED FAT 2.1G
TRANS FAT 0.0G **SODIUM** 865MG **TOTAL CARBOHYDRATES** 65.3G **SUGARS** 12.2G **PROTEIN** 14.2G

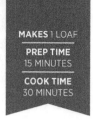
Grain-Free Sandwich Bread

This sandwich bread is made without any grains at all. Almond flour gives it a hearty dose of protein and healthy fat. Simple and delicious, it's great for everyday sandwiches, like turkey or ham and cheese. It's also great toasted and spread with goat cheese or honey.

NONSTICK COOKING SPRAY

1½ CUPS ALMOND FLOUR

¾ CUP ARROWROOT POWDER

¼ CUP GOLDEN FLAXSEED MEAL

½ TEASPOON SALT

½ TEASPOON BAKING SODA

4 EGGS

1 TEASPOON HONEY

1 TEASPOON APPLE CIDER VINEGAR

1. Preheat the oven to 350°F.

2. Spray a standard-size loaf pan with the cooking spray.

3. In a medium bowl, stir together the almond flour, arrowroot, flaxseed meal, salt, and baking soda.

4. Using an electric hand mixer in a large bowl or in the bowl of your stand mixer, beat the eggs until they are foamy. Add the honey and vinegar to the eggs, then add the dry ingredients and mix well.

5. Transfer the batter to the prepared loaf pan and smooth the top with a spatula or the back of a spoon.

6. Bake the bread until it is golden brown and a toothpick inserted into the center comes out clean, about 30 minutes.

7. Cool the bread on a wire rack before slicing.

NUTRITIONAL INFORMATION PER SLICE (12 SLICES PER LOAF): CALORIES 88 TOTAL FAT 4.0G SATURATED FAT 0.7G TRANS FAT 0.0G SODIUM 171MG TOTAL CARBOHYDRATES 10.0G SUGARS 0.7G PROTEIN 11.3G

GRAIN-FREE SANDWICH BREAD RECIPE

Chicken Salad Sandwiches with Arugula

Peppery arugula adds a nice bite to this vinaigrette-dressed chicken salad with salty feta cheese. This sandwich is a great way to use up leftover rotisserie or homemade roasted chicken. You could also substitute roasted turkey if you're looking for a way to use up Thanksgiving leftovers.

2 TABLESPOONS EXTRA-VIRGIN OLIVE OIL

1 TABLESPOON RED WINE VINEGAR

1 TEASPOON FRESH OR DRIED ROSEMARY, CRUSHED

½ TEASPOON DRIED OREGANO

¼ TEASPOON SALT

¼ TEASPOON CRUSHED RED PEPPER

2 CUPS DICED COOKED CHICKEN BREAST

¼ CUP FINELY CHOPPED RED ONION

6 TABLESPOONS CRUMBLED FETA CHEESE

8 SLICES GRAIN-FREE SANDWICH BREAD, LIGHTLY TOASTED

1 TOMATO, CUT INTO 4 SLICES

2 CUPS PACKED ARUGULA

1. In a medium bowl, combine the olive oil, vinegar, rosemary, oregano, salt, and red pepper, and whisk to emulsify.

2. Stir in the chicken, onion, and feta cheese, and mix gently until well combined.

3. Divide the chicken mixture evenly among 4 slices of the toasted bread. Top each with a tomato slice and ½ cup of the arugula. Place the remaining toast slices on top of the sandwiches.

4. Cut each sandwich in half diagonally and serve immediately.

NUTRITIONAL INFORMATION PER SERVING: CALORIES 391 TOTAL FAT 16.9G SATURATED FAT 3.1G
TRANS FAT 0.0G SODIUM 575MG TOTAL CARBOHYDRATES 38.6G SUGARS 3.5G PROTEIN 32.6G

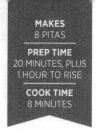

MAKES
8 PITAS

PREP TIME
20 MINUTES, PLUS
1 HOUR TO RISE

COOK TIME
8 MINUTES

Pita Bread

This simple pocket bread is easy to make. If you have one, a pizza stone works especially well for baking light, airy pitas.

3 TO 4½ CUPS GLUTEN-FREE
   ALL-PURPOSE FLOUR
2 TEASPOONS XANTHAN GUM
1 TEASPOON SALT
4 TEASPOONS ACTIVE DRY YEAST

3 TABLESPOONS SUGAR
3 TABLESPOONS CANOLA OIL, PLUS
   MORE FOR THE BOWL
2½ CUPS WARM WHOLE OR LOW-FAT
   (NOT NONFAT) MILK

1. Using an electric hand mixer in a large bowl or in the bowl of your stand mixer, combine 3 cups of flour, the xanthan gum, and the salt, and mix well.

2. Add the yeast, sugar, and canola oil one at a time, mixing after each addition.

3. With the mixer set to low speed, drizzle in the milk in a thin stream. Continue to mix until the dough comes together. If necessary, add additional flour, ¼ cup at a time, until the dough is thick and tacky.

4. Transfer the dough to a large, oiled bowl. Turn it over to coat, cover it with plastic wrap, and set it in a warm place to rise for about 1 hour. The dough should just about double in size.

5. Preheat the oven to 475°F.

6. Sprinkle your work surface generously with flour. Split the dough into 8 equal portions and coat each lightly with flour. Working with one piece of dough at a time, flatten it with the heel of your hand and then your fingertips to make a smooth, flat, airless round about 6 inches across.

7. Place the rounds on a pizza stone or baking sheet, arranging them so they don't touch. Bake until the rounds puff up, about 6 to 8 minutes.

8. Remove the pitas from the oven and allow them to cool before using.

NUTRITIONAL INFORMATION PER PITA: CALORIES 341 TOTAL FAT 6.1G SATURATED FAT 0.9G
TRANS FAT 0.0G SODIUM 355MG TOTAL CARBOHYDRATES 61.1G SUGARS 10.5G PROTEIN 7.3G

Greek Salad in a Pita

SERVES 4

PREP TIME
10 MINUTES

Homemade pita bread makes a great edible serving plate for a tangy and crisp Greek salad. This version has the classic diced cucumber, tomato, red onion, Kalamata olives, and crumbled feta cheese, plus a handful of diced radishes for extra crunch. You can add or subtract vegetables according to what you like and what's fresh at the market at the moment.

3 TABLESPOONS EXTRA-VIRGIN OLIVE OIL

1 TABLESPOON RED WINE VINEGAR

1 TEASPOON CRUMBLED DRIED OREGANO

½ TEASPOON SALT

¼ TEASPOON FRESHLY GROUND BLACK PEPPER

1¼ CUPS CHOPPED, SEEDED PLUM OR CHERRY TOMATOES

1 CUP PEELED, SEEDED, AND DICED CUCUMBER

1 CUP DICED GREEN OR RED BELL PEPPER

⅔ CUP DICED RED ONION

½ CUP DICED RADISHES

⅓ CUP CHOPPED, PITTED KALAMATA OLIVES

½ CUP CHOPPED FRESH ITALIAN PARSLEY

1 CUP CRUMBLED FETA CHEESE

4 PITA ROUNDS, HALVED

1. In a large bowl, whisk together the olive oil, vinegar, oregano, salt, and black pepper to emulsify.

2. Add the tomatoes, cucumber, bell pepper, onion, radishes, olives, and parsley, and stir to combine. Gently fold in the feta cheese.

3. Divide the salad into 8 portions. Open each pita half and, using a slotted spoon, scoop in a portion of the salad mixture.

4. Serve immediately, 2 pita halves to a plate.

NUTRITIONAL INFORMATION PER SERVING: CALORIES 444 TOTAL FAT 24.2G SATURATED FAT 7.4G TRANS FAT 0.0G
SODIUM 1,423MG TOTAL CARBOHYDRATES 48.8G SUGARS 8.6G PROTEIN 12.9G

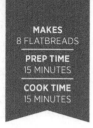

MAKES
8 FLATBREADS

PREP TIME
15 MINUTES

COOK TIME
15 MINUTES

Grain-Free Flatbread

Made with a nutritious blend of coconut and almond flour, this soft, chewy flatbread makes a great base for pizza. It's also ideal for cutting into wedges to use as dippers for hummus, baba ghanoush, and other dips.

⅞ CUP SIFTED COCONUT FLOUR

¼ CUP PSYLLIUM HUSK POWDER

2 TABLESPOONS ALMOND FLOUR

½ CUP COCONUT OIL, MELTED

½ TEASPOON SALT

1 TEASPOON HONEY OR SUGAR

2 CUPS HOT WATER

GRAPESEED OR COCONUT OIL,
    FOR FRYING

1. In a large bowl, whisk together the coconut flour, psyllium husk powder, and almond flour. Stir in the melted coconut oil, salt, and honey until well combined.

2. Break the dough up and then pour the hot water over it. Stir until the clumps of dough and liquid are completely incorporated.

3. Divide the dough into 8 equal portions and shape each into a ball. Using the heel of your hand, flatten each ball into a disk, then use your fingertips to flatten it further.

4. Lay a piece of parchment paper on your work surface and place one dough disk on it at a time. Cover each with a second piece of parchment paper and use a rolling pin to flatten each disk into a 6- or 7-inch round. Repeat with all the disks.

5. Coat a large, heavy skillet lightly with oil and heat it over medium heat. Place one flatbread at a time in the skillet and cook until it is nicely browned on the bottom and beginning to puff up, 5 to 7 minutes. Flip the flatbread over and cook the second side until is browned, another 5 to 7 minutes. Repeat with the remaining flatbreads.

NUTRITIONAL INFORMATION PER FLATBREAD: CALORIES 222   TOTAL FAT 18.6G   SATURATED FAT 12.5G
TRANS FAT 0.0G   SODIUM 182MG   TOTAL CARBOHYDRATES 10.2G   SUGARS 2.0G   PROTEIN 3.5G

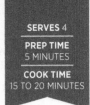
GRAIN-FREE FLATBREAD RECIPE

Flatbread with Goat Cheese, Figs, and Prosciutto

These flatbreads, topped with creamy goat cheese, sweet figs, and salty prosciutto, are like highly refined little pizzas. The prosciutto is optional; this dish is just as delicious when made vegetarian. Don't skip the balsamic reduction, however, because it is what makes this recipe shine.

4 GRAIN-FREE FLATBREADS
⅔ CUP BALSAMIC VINEGAR
12 OUNCES FRESH GOAT CHEESE
8 RIPE BLACK MISSION FIGS, SLICED

6 OUNCES PROSCIUTTO, VERY THINLY SLICED
2 CUPS ARUGULA

1. Preheat the oven to 425°F.

2. Place 4 flatbread rounds on a large baking sheet.

3. In a small saucepan set over medium-low heat, add the vinegar and bring it to a simmer. Let the vinegar simmer, stirring occasionally, until it becomes thick and syrupy, about 10 minutes. Set aside to cool.

4. Crumble the goat cheese onto the flatbread rounds, dividing evenly among the 4 flatbreads. Add the sliced figs, dividing evenly.

5. Bake the flatbreads about 6 to 8 minutes, until the cheese is bubbly and the figs have begun to soften.

6. Divide the prosciutto evenly over the flatbreads and then top each with ½ cup of arugula.

7. Drizzle the reduced balsamic vinegar evenly over the top of each flatbread. Serve immediately.

NUTRITIONAL INFORMATION PER SERVING: CALORIES 622 TOTAL FAT 35.5G SATURATED FAT 21.8G TRANS FAT 0.0G SODIUM 1,022MG TOTAL CARBOHYDRATES 38.5G SUGARS 18.5G PROTEIN 44.9G

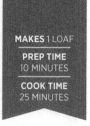
Rosemary and Garlic Focaccia

This grain-free focaccia will satisfy your cravings for this popular olive-oil-infused bread. Made with a combination of flaxseed meal and almond flour and spiked with plenty of garlic, rosemary, and crushed red pepper flakes, it's delicious all on its own, but don't let that stop you from dunking it in balsamic vinegar or topping it with a flavorful cheese. It also makes a great base for a quick pizza.

NONSTICK COOKING SPRAY

1 CUP GOLDEN FLAXSEED MEAL

1 CUP ALMOND FLOUR

1½ TABLESPOONS BAKING POWDER

1 TABLESPOON MINCED FRESH
    ROSEMARY

1 TEASPOON CRUSHED RED
    PEPPER FLAKES

½ TEASPOON SALT

8 EGGS, LIGHTLY BEATEN

¼ CUP EXTRA-VIRGIN OLIVE OIL

4 GARLIC CLOVES, MINCED

½ TEASPOON COARSE SALT, FOR
    SPRINKLING

1. Preheat the oven to 350°F.

2. Spray a 9-inch-square baking pan with cooking spray.

3. In a medium bowl, whisk together the flaxseed meal, almond flour, baking powder, rosemary, red pepper flakes, and salt. Stir in the eggs, olive oil, and garlic, and mix until well incorporated.

4. Scrape the batter into the prepared pan and smooth out the top. Sprinkle the salt over the top.

5. Bake the bread until it is puffed and golden brown, about 25 minutes.

6. Cool the bread in the pan on a wire rack before slicing.

NUTRITIONAL INFORMATION PER SLICE (6 SLICES PER LOAF): CALORIES 273 TOTAL FAT 22.8G SATURATED FAT 4.0G TRANS FAT 0.0G SODIUM 442MG TOTAL CARBOHYDRATES 9.7G SUGARS 0.0G PROTEIN 12.6G

ROSEMARY AND GARLIC FOCACCIA RECIPE

Vegetable and Cheese Sandwich on Herbed Focaccia

This herbed bread makes a wonderful snack or appetizer all by itself. To elevate it to an amazing sandwich, a few fillings are all you need. This sandwich is heavenly in its simplicity—a mild cheese, an assortment of fresh veggies, and a dash of balsamic vinegar and good olive oil.

1 ROSEMARY AND GARLIC
    FOCACCIA LOAF
6 OUNCES PROVOLONE OR HAVARTI
    CHEESE, THINLY SLICED
12 (¼-INCH-THICK) TOMATO SLICES
½ CUP CHOPPED SCALLIONS
4 CUPS MIXED SALAD GREENS

3 TABLESPOONS BALSAMIC VINEGAR
2 TABLESPOONS EXTRA-VIRGIN
    OLIVE OIL
½ TEASPOON SALT
¼ TEASPOON FRESHLY GROUND
    BLACK PEPPER

1. Using a large serrated knife, slice the whole focaccia loaf in half horizontally. Arrange the cheese and tomato slices in an even layer over the bottom half of the bread. Sprinkle the scallions over the tomatoes, then top them with the salad greens.

2. In a small bowl, whisk together the vinegar, olive oil, salt, and pepper. Drizzle the dressing over the bottom half of the sandwich.

3. Place the top half of the focaccia over the filling and cut the sandwich loaf into 6 portions. Serve immediately.

NUTRITIONAL INFORMATION PER SERVING: CALORIES 435 TOTAL FAT 35.1G SATURATED FAT 9.5G
TRANS FAT 0.0G SODIUM 911MG TOTAL CARBOHYDRATES 14.8G SUGARS 0.9G PROTEIN 21.4G

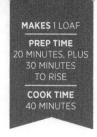

MAKES 1 LOAF

PREP TIME
20 MINUTES, PLUS
30 MINUTES
TO RISE

COOK TIME
40 MINUTES

Cinnamon Bread

Slightly sweet cinnamon bread makes a great quick breakfast, and a surprisingly good sandwich with savory fillings such as creamy goat cheese, and herby greens.

BUTTER, FOR GREASING THE PAN

1 CUP BROWN RICE FLOUR

¾ CUP WHITE RICE FLOUR

½ CUP POTATO STARCH

¼ CUP TAPIOCA STARCH

2 TABLESPOONS SUGAR

2½ TEASPOONS XANTHAN GUM

2 TEASPOONS RAPID-RISE YEAST

1½ TEASPOONS SALT

1 CUP MILK

2 TEASPOONS APPLE CIDER VINEGAR

2 TABLESPOONS VEGETABLE OIL

3 EGGS

½ CUP POWDERED SUGAR

1½ TABLESPOONS GROUND CINNAMON

½ TEASPOON VANILLA EXTRACT

2 TO 3 TEASPOONS WATER

1. Preheat the oven to 350°F. Butter a standard-size loaf pan.

2. In a small bowl, whisk together the rice flours, potato starch, tapioca starch, sugar, xanthan gum, yeast, and 1¼ teaspoons of salt.

3. Using an electric hand mixer in a large bowl or in the bowl of your stand mixer, stir together the milk, vinegar, vegetable oil, and eggs. Add the dry ingredients and mix for 3 minutes with the mixer set on medium speed, until the batter is smooth.

4. In a small bowl, combine the powdered sugar, cinnamon, vanilla, remaining ¼ teaspoon of salt, and water; start with 2 teaspoons of water and add more if needed to make a smooth paste.

5. Swirl half the cinnamon mixture into the batter and fold it in using a spatula. Repeat with the remaining cinnamon mixture. Be careful not to over mix.

6. Transfer the dough to the prepared loaf pan and let it rise in a warm spot for about 30 minutes, until the dough rises to the top of the sides of the pan.

7. Bake the bread until the top is golden brown, 35 to 40 minutes. Run a knife around the edge of the pan to release the loaf and transfer it to a wire rack to cool before slicing.

NUTRITIONAL INFORMATION PER SLICE (12 SLICES PER LOAF):   CALORIES 204   TOTAL FAT 4.3G   SATURATED FAT 1.1G   TRANS FAT 0.0G   SODIUM 318MG   TOTAL CARBOHYDRATES 37.2G   SUGARS 8.2G   PROTEIN 3.5G

CINNAMON BREAD RECIPE

Cinnamon-Apple Grilled Cheese

This sandwich delivers the crave-worthy combination of sweet and salty flavors with the slightly sweet bread and salty Cheddar cheese. Crisp green apple adds an acidic punch, along with a welcome bit of crunch. This grilled sandwich would be equally at home on your brunch or lunch table.

8 SLICES SHARP WHITE
CHEDDAR CHEESE

8 SLICES CINNAMON BREAD

1 LARGE GRANNY SMITH APPLE, PEELED, CORED, AND THINLY SLICED

NONSTICK COOKING SPRAY

1. Divide the Cheddar cheese equally among 4 slices of bread. Top the cheese with the apple slices. Place the remaining 4 bread slices on top of the sandwiches.

2. Spray a skillet or panini press with nonstick cooking spray and heat it to medium-high. When the pan is hot, reduce the heat to medium and place the sandwiches in the pan.

3. If using a skillet, cover the pan and cook for about 4 minutes, until the underside is nicely browned. Flip the sandwich over, cover again, and cook until the second side is browned and the cheese is melted, another 4 minutes. If using a panini press, close the press and cook until both sides are nicely browned and the cheese is melted, about 5 minutes total.

4. Serve immediately.

NUTRITIONAL INFORMATION PER SERVING: CALORIES 667 TOTAL FAT 27.5G SATURATED FAT 14.2G TRANS FAT 0.0G SODIUM 989MG TOTAL CARBOHYDRATES 82.8G SUGARS 22.5G PROTEIN 21.1G

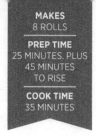

MAKES
8 ROLLS

PREP TIME
25 MINUTES, PLUS
45 MINUTES
TO RISE

COOK TIME
35 MINUTES

Pretzel Rolls

On their own these salty rolls are a delicious snack, but they also make great sandwich rolls. Unsalted butter, egg whites, and water should be room temperature.

3¼ CUPS GLUTEN-FREE
    ALL-PURPOSE FLOUR

1½ TEASPOONS XANTHAN GUM

½ CUP CULTURED BUTTERMILK
    POWDER OR DRY MILK POWDER

1 TABLESPOON INSTANT DRY YEAST

¼ TEASPOON CREAM OF TARTAR

1 TABLESPOON LIGHT BROWN SUGAR

1¼ TEASPOON BAKING SODA, DIVIDED

2 TEASPOONS SALT, DIVIDED

1 TEASPOON APPLE CIDER VINEGAR

2 TABLESPOONS UNSALTED BUTTER

2 EGG WHITES

1½ CUPS LUKEWARM WATER

6 CUPS WATER

COARSE SALT, FOR SPRINKLING

1. Line a baking sheet with parchment paper.

2. Using a mixer of your choice, whisk together the flour, xanthan gum, buttermilk powder, yeast, cream of tartar, brown sugar, and ¼ teaspoon of baking soda. Add 1 teaspoon of salt, vinegar, butter, and egg whites, and beat on medium speed until well combined.

3. With the mixer on low, drizzle in the lukewarm water. Beat on high speed for 3 minutes. If necessary, add additional flour, 1 tablespoon at a time, and mix on low until the dough is wet but starting to pull away from the sides of the bowl.

4. Transfer dough to a lightly floured work surface and sprinkle with a bit more flour. Divide dough into 8 equal portions and shape each into a round disk. Place each disk onto the prepared baking sheet.

5. Loosely cover the baking sheet with plastic wrap and let the dough rise in a warm spot for about 45 minutes. The balls should double in size. Preheat the oven to 375°F.

6. In a medium stockpot, combine 6 cups of water with remaining baking soda and salt. Bring to a boil. Drop the dough disks into the boiling solution, 2 or 3 at a time. After about 1 minute, remove with a slotted spoon and place on the parchment-lined baking sheet.

7. Make several shallow parallel slashes in the top of each disk, sprinkle them with coarse salt, and bake them for about 30 minutes, until they are golden brown.

NUTRITIONAL INFORMATION PER ROLL: CALORIES 302 TOTAL FAT 2.9 SATURATED FAT 1.8G TRANS FAT 0.0G
SODIUM 432MG TOTAL CARBOHYDRATES 57.6G SUGARS 5.5G PROTEIN 8.3G

PRETZEL ROLLS RECIPE

Leftover Holiday Ham Sandwiches with Hot-Sweet Mustard

These simple sandwiches—sweet-salty glazed ham nestled into chewy pretzel rolls and spread with tangy hot-sweet mustard—are the best way to use up a leftover holiday ham. Serve them with an ice-cold gluten-free beer (for the grown-ups, of course), and you've got yourself a near perfect meal.

3 TABLESPOONS HOT-SWEET MUSTARD
   (SUCH AS HONEY-DIJON)
4 PRETZEL ROLLS, SPLIT

10 OUNCES BAKED HAM, SLICED
2 CUPS ARUGULA

1. Spread the mustard onto the rolls, dividing evenly.

2. Divide the ham and arugula into four portions and fill each roll.

3. Serve immediately.

NUTRITIONAL INFORMATION PER SERVING: CALORIES 392 TOTAL FAT 4.8G SATURATED FAT 1.8G
TRANS FAT 0.0G SODIUM 1,322MG TOTAL CARBOHYDRATES 58.5G SUGARS 5.5G PROTEIN 21.9G

MAKES
8 ROLLS

PREP TIME
20 MINUTES, PLUS
40 MINUTES
TO RISE

COOK TIME
45 MINUTES

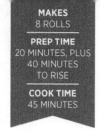

Hoagie Rolls

When you're in the mood for a hoagie (or grinder or sub, depending on where you live), you'll want to have one of these on hand. Fill it with meatballs, eggplant parmesan, or tuna salad, or just load it up with your favorite sandwich fixings.

¼ CUP CORNMEAL, FOR DUSTING

2 TABLESPOONS SUGAR

1½ CUPS LUKEWARM WATER

2 TABLESPOONS INSTANT DRY YEAST

2 CUPS WHITE RICE FLOUR

½ CUP TAPIOCA STARCH

½ CUP POTATO STARCH

3 TEASPOONS XANTHAN GUM

1½ TEASPOONS SALT

2 TABLESPOONS UNSALTED
   BUTTER, MELTED

3 EGG WHITES, LIGHTLY BEATEN

1 TEASPOON WHITE VINEGAR

1. Dust 2 large baking sheets with cornmeal.

2. In a small bowl, stir the sugar into the warm water, then stir in the yeast. Let the mixture sit for 5 to 10 minutes, until it becomes frothy.

3. Using a mixer of your choice, combine the rice flour, tapioca starch, potato starch, xanthan gum, and salt. Turn mixer on low and mix to combine.

4. Add the yeast mixture and mix to combine.

5. Add the butter, egg whites, and vinegar. With the mixer on high speed, beat for about 3 minutes.

6. Form the mixture into 8 rolls and set them several inches apart on the baking sheets. Make several diagonal slashes in the top of each roll. Cover rolls with plastic wrap and let them rise in a warm place for 25 to 30 minutes, until they double in size.

7. Preheat the oven to 400°F.

8. Bake the rolls for about 45 minutes, until they are golden brown and cooked through. Let the rolls cool on a wire rack before slicing.

NUTRITIONAL INFORMATION PER ROLL: CALORIES 288   TOTAL FAT 3.6G   SATURATED FAT 1.8G
TRANS FAT 0.0G   SODIUM 482MG   TOTAL CARBOHYDRATES 57.8G   SUGARS 3.4G   PROTEIN 3.7G

Authentic Italian Meat and Cheese Hoagies

SERVES 4

PREP TIME
10 MINUTES

These Italian-style submarine sandwiches are popular on the East Coast. They make a great game-day lunch. The sliced hot peppers are what make these sandwiches extra special, but if you don't like that much heat, substitute milder peppers such as peperoncini. If you're planning to pack them for later, leave off the dressing, which will make the sandwich soggy. Bring it along in a small jar or plastic container and drizzle on the dressing just before eating.

4 HOAGIE ROLLS, SPLIT HORIZONTALLY

12 SLICES HARD SALAMI

12 THIN SLICES CAPICOLA OR
     DELI HAM

8 THIN SLICES PROVOLONE CHEESE

1 WHITE ONION, THINLY SLICED

12 THIN SLICES TOMATO

1½ CUPS FINELY SHREDDED LETTUCE

¼ CUP EXTRA-VIRGIN OLIVE OIL

2 TABLESPOONS RED WINE VINEGAR

1 TEASPOON DRIED OREGANO

4 BOTTLED HOT CHERRY PEPPERS,
     THINLY SLICED

SALT (OPTIONAL)

FRESHLY GROUND BLACK PEPPER
     (OPTIONAL)

1. Layer the bottom half of the rolls with the salami, capicola, provolone cheese, onion, and tomato. Top each with lettuce.

2. In a small bowl, whisk together the olive oil, vinegar, oregano, and sliced peppers. Taste and add salt and pepper (if using).

3. Drizzle the dressing over the fillings, then top with the top half of the rolls.

4. Cut each sandwich in half and serve immediately.

NUTRITIONAL INFORMATION PER SERVING: CALORIES 792 **TOTAL FAT** 43.5G **SATURATED FAT** 14.6G
TRANS FAT 0.0G **SODIUM** 2,915MG **TOTAL CARBOHYDRATES** 67.8G **SUGARS** 5.4G **PROTEIN** 30.3G

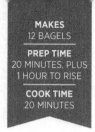

MAKES
12 BAGELS

PREP TIME
20 MINUTES, PLUS
1 HOUR TO RISE

COOK TIME
20 MINUTES

Bagels

With these delicious bagels, you'll never feel deprived—so make a double batch. When the bagels are cool, slice a bunch and freeze them in plastic bags.

2 PACKETS RAPID-RISE YEAST

2 CUPS WARM WATER

5½ CUPS GLUTEN-FREE
   ALL-PURPOSE FLOUR

3 TABLESPOONS SUGAR

2 TEASPOONS SALT

NONSTICK COOKING SPRAY

2 QUARTS WATER

2 TEASPOONS CANOLA OIL

1. In a small bowl, stir together the yeast and warm water. Let it sit for 5 to 10 minutes, until frothy.

2. Using an electric hand mixer in a large bowl or in the bowl of your stand mixer fitted with the dough hook, mix together the flour, sugar, and salt. Add the yeast mixture and mix on medium speed until the dough is smooth.

3. Cover the dough with plastic wrap and let it rise for 10 minutes.

4. Divide the dough into 12 equal portions. Roll each piece between the palms of your hands to make a rope. Press the ends of the rope together to make a ring, using a bit of water if needed to make the two ends stick together.

5. Place the bagels a few inches apart on a baking sheet, cover them with plastic wrap, and let them rise for about 45 minutes, until they have expanded by about half.

6. Preheat the oven to 400°F. Spray a large baking sheet with cooking spray.

7. In a large stockpot, combine the water with the canola oil and bring to a boil. Drop the bagels, two or three at a time, into the boiling water for about 45 seconds. Turn each bagel over with a slotted spoon and cook for 45 seconds more. Remove the bagels from the water with the slotted spoon and place them on the prepared baking sheet.

8. Bake the bagels until they turn a nice golden brown on top, about 18 minutes. Remove the baking sheet from the oven and let the bagels cool on it before slicing.

NUTRITIONAL INFORMATION PER BAGEL: CALORIES 385   TOTAL FAT 0.8G   SATURATED FAT 0.0G
TRANS FAT 0.0G   SODIUM 814MG   TOTAL CARBOHYDRATES 87.3G   SUGARS 3.0G   PROTEIN 3.6G

BAGELS RECIPE

Bagels and Lox

Bagels and lox are a classic Sunday-morning combo. The addition of capers and chives makes this sandwich worthy of any special occasion. Lox is brined, cold-smoked salmon. There are many variations on this idea, from nova lox to Scottish salmon, and all will be delicious here.

4 BAGELS, CUT IN HALF
    HORIZONTALLY
8 OUNCES WHIPPED CREAM CHEESE
¼ CUP DRAINED CAPERS
8 OUNCES SLICED LOX

⅓ CUP THINLY SLICED RED ONION
2 TABLESPOONS MINCED CHIVES,
    FOR GARNISH
FRESHLY GROUND BLACK PEPPER

1. Spread 4 bagel halves with cream cheese.

2. Sprinkle on the capers and top each bagel half with a slice of lox.

3. Arrange the red onion slices on top, garnish with the chives, and grind a bit of pepper over the tops.

4. Serve immediately.

NUTRITIONAL INFORMATION PER SERVING: CALORIES 594   TOTAL FAT 4.1G   SATURATED FAT 1.1G
TRANS FAT 0.0G   SODIUM 2,512MG   TOTAL CARBOHYDRATES 92.4G   SUGARS 3.9G   PROTEIN 22.5G

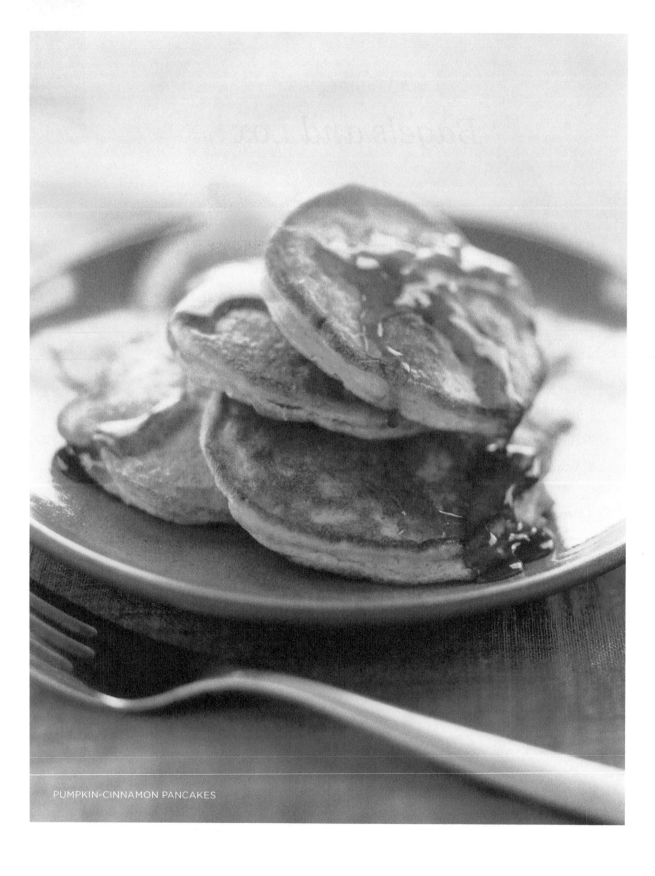

PUMPKIN-CINNAMON PANCAKES

5

Breakfasts

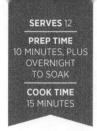

SERVES 12

PREP TIME
10 MINUTES, PLUS
OVERNIGHT
TO SOAK

COOK TIME
15 MINUTES

Cranberry Granola

Cereal is a quick and easy breakfast that's perfect for busy weekdays, but many of the old standbys contain gluten. This sweet and crunchy granola is full of protein and fiber, so it will keep you satisfied all morning, and it's gluten-free. Serve it with milk or sprinkled over yogurt. You can even use it as a delicious topping for a baked fruit crumble.

Time-saving tip This granola keeps well in an airtight container in your pantry. Mix up a big batch and keep it on hand for quick breakfasts and healthy snacks. For variety, substitute different nuts, seeds, or dried fruits, as desired.

2 CUPS WHOLE SHELLED ALMONDS

1 CUP WALNUT HALVES

1 CUP SHELLED PUMPKIN SEEDS

NONSTICK COOKING SPRAY

1 CUP DRIED CRANBERRIES

1 CUP WATER

1 TABLESPOON VANILLA EXTRACT

½ TEASPOON GROUND CINNAMON

½ TEASPOON SALT

2 TABLESPOONS HONEY

1. Combine the almonds, walnuts, and pumpkin seeds in a bowl, and cover them with water. Soak overnight.

2. Preheat the oven to 350°F.

3. Spray 2 baking sheets with nonstick cooking spray.

4. Place the cranberries in a food processor or blender with the water and purée until smooth.

5. Drain the almond mixture, then add it to the food processor or blender with the cranberries. Pulse until the mixture is coarsely chopped.

6. Transfer the mixture to a medium bowl and stir in the vanilla, cinnamon, and salt.

7. Spread the granola in a thin layer on the prepared baking sheets. Drizzle the granola with the honey.

8. Bake the granola for 15 minutes, or until it is lightly toasted.

9. Serve the granola warm or at room temperature.

10. Store the granola at room temperature in an airtight container.

NUTRITIONAL INFORMATION PER SERVING: CALORIES 186   TOTAL FAT 15.0G   SATURATED FAT 1.5G
TRANS FAT 0.0G   SODIUM 100MG   TOTAL CARBOHYDRATES 8.6G   SUGARS 3.7G   PROTEIN 6.7G

Pumpkin Coconut Breakfast Porridge

Chia seeds, when combined with hot water, act as a thickening agent, making this porridge especially hearty. Quick to make and loaded with nuts and seeds, this hot cereal really packs a nutritional punch. Breakfast doesn't get much better.

Ingredient tip Make sure you get pumpkin purée—nothing but pumpkin. Pumpkin pie filling has added sweeteners and flavorings.

⅓ CUP CHOPPED WALNUTS

3 TABLESPOONS UNSWEETENED
    FLAKED COCONUT

2 TABLESPOONS TOASTED
    SESAME SEEDS

2 TABLESPOONS WHOLE FLAXSEED

2 TABLESPOONS CHIA SEEDS

1 TABLESPOON PUMPKIN PURÉE

1½ TEASPOONS GROUND CINNAMON

PINCH SALT

2 CUPS BOILING WATER

1. In a blender, combine the walnuts, coconut, sesame seeds, flaxseed, chia seeds, pumpkin purée, cinnamon, and salt, and blend until smooth.

2. Add the boiling water and blend on low until well combined, then turn to high speed and blend until smooth, about 30 seconds.

3. Pour the porridge into 2 bowls and serve hot.

NUTRITIONAL INFORMATION PER SERVING: CALORIES 397 TOTAL FAT 35.9G SATURATED FAT 4.6G
TRANS FAT 0.0G SODIUM 86MG TOTAL CARBOHYDRATES 18.4G SUGARS 1.1G PROTEIN 15.0G

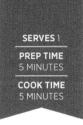
Mushroom and Egg White Omelet

Made with egg whites rather than whole eggs, this omelet is low in fat and cholesterol but high in protein. Enjoy it with a thick slice of toasted gluten-free bread. Substitute fresh thyme for the chives if you want a bit of variety; it pairs perfectly with earthy mushrooms.

Time-saving tip Many supermarkets carry sliced fresh mushrooms. Since chopping mushrooms is the majority of the prep for this dish, buying them already cut is a real time-saver.

1 TEASPOON EXTRA VIRGIN OLIVE OIL

4 EGG WHITES

½ TEASPOON SALT

1 TABLESPOON CHOPPED
    FRESH CHIVES

½ CUP DICED MUSHROOMS

1 TABLESPOON FRESHLY GRATED
    PARMESAN CHEESE, FOR GARNISH

1. Heat the olive oil in a small skillet over low heat.

2. In a small bowl, beat together the egg whites, salt, and chives.

3. Pour the egg mixture into the skillet and tilt to spread the eggs. Stir gently with a spatula while cooking for about 1 minute.

4. Let the egg cook without stirring for 1 minute, then sprinkle it with the mushrooms.

5. Run the spatula along the edges of the skillet, loosening the cooked egg and allowing the uncooked egg to flow underneath.

6. Cook the omelet until the egg is almost set, about 3 more minutes, then fold half the omelet over the other half.

7. Lightly press down on the omelet with the spatula and slide it onto a plate.

8. Garnish the omelet with Parmesan cheese and serve hot.

NUTRITIONAL INFORMATION PER SERVING: CALORIES 202 TOTAL FAT 11.2G SATURATED FAT 4.7G
TRANS FAT 0.0G SODIUM 1,645MG TOTAL CARBOHYDRATES 3.1G SUGARS 1.5G PROTEIN 24.6G

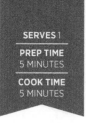
Tomato, Basil, and Egg White Omelet

Make this omelet in the summertime when tomatoes are at their peak. Loaded with bright tomato flavor and herby basil and kept light by leaving out the yolks, this omelet is sure to wake you up and keep you going throughout the morning.

Ingredient tip Don't waste those yolks! Egg yolks freeze well if you beat in a pinch of salt or a bit of sugar before popping them in the freezer (add ⅛ teaspoon of salt or 1½ teaspoons of sugar for every 4 yolks). Store them in a well-marked container (be sure to note if you've added salt or sugar) and pull them out the next time you want to whip up a cake, pudding, or rich pasta sauce like Alfredo.

1 TEASPOON EXTRA-VIRGIN OLIVE OIL

4 EGG WHITES

½ TEASPOON SALT

1 TABLESPOON CHOPPED FRESH BASIL

1 TOMATO, DICED

1 TABLESPOON FRESHLY GRATED
PARMESAN CHEESE, FOR GARNISH

1. Heat the olive oil in a small skillet over low heat.

2. In a small bowl, beat together the egg whites, salt, and basil.

3. Pour the egg mixture into the skillet and tilt to spread the eggs. Stir gently with a spatula while cooking for about 1 minute.

4. Let the egg cook without stirring for 1 minute, then sprinkle it with the tomato.

5. Run the spatula along the edges of the skillet, loosening the cooked egg and allowing the uncooked egg to flow underneath.

6. Cook the omelet until the egg is almost set, then fold half the omelet over the other half.

7. Lightly press down on the omelet with the spatula and slide it onto a plate.

8. Garnish the omelet with the Parmesan cheese and serve hot.

NUTRITIONAL INFORMATION PER SERVING: CALORIES 206 CALORIES FROM FAT: 44 **TOTAL FAT** 11.2 **SATURATED FAT** 4.7G
TRANS FAT 0.0G **SODIUM** 1,646MG **TOTAL CARBOHYDRATES** 4.6G **SUGARS** 2.4G **PROTEIN** 24.0G

Ham and Cheese Frittata

SERVES 4

PREP TIME
10 MINUTES

COOK TIME
20 MINUTES

Made with diced ham and Cheddar cheese, this frittata is likely to be a big hit with the little ones. Frittata is just as good at room temperature as it is warm from the oven, so consider making up a pan of this on the weekend and packing the leftovers into lunchboxes throughout the week.

9 EGGS

2 TABLESPOONS FAT-FREE MILK

1 TEASPOON SALT

3 TABLESPOONS FRESHLY GRATED
    PARMESAN CHEESE

1 TABLESPOON EXTRA-VIRGIN OLIVE OIL

¼ CUP DICED YELLOW ONION

1 GARLIC CLOVE, MINCED

1 CUP DICED HAM

¾ CUP SHREDDED CHEDDAR CHEESE

1. Preheat the oven to 400°F.

2. In a medium bowl, whisk together the eggs, milk, salt, and Parmesan cheese. Set aside.

3. Heat the olive oil in a medium ovenproof skillet over medium heat. Add the onion and garlic and cook, stirring frequently, for 4 minutes, or until the onions are translucent.

4. Add the ham and cook for 1 minute, stirring often.

5. Spread the mixture evenly in the skillet, then pour the egg mixture over it.

6. Sprinkle the frittata with ½ cup of Cheddar cheese.

7. Let the frittata cook for 5 minutes, undisturbed, until halfway set, then transfer the skillet, uncovered, to the oven.

8. Bake for 8 to 10 minutes, until the frittata is puffed. Sprinkle the frittata with the remaining ¼ cup of Cheddar and cook for 2 minutes more, or until the cheese is melted.

9. Remove the frittata from the oven and let it sit for 5 minutes.

10. Serve the frittata hot or at room temperature, cut into wedges.

NUTRITIONAL INFORMATION PER SERVING: CALORIES 386   TOTAL FAT 27.8G   SATURATED FAT 12.0G
TRANS FAT 0.0G   SODIUM 1,491MG   TOTAL CARBOHYDRATES 4.4G   SUGARS 1.6G   PROTEIN 30.4G

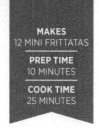

MAKES
12 MINI FRITTATAS

PREP TIME
10 MINUTES

COOK TIME
25 MINUTES

Mini Sausage Frittatas

Made in muffin tins, these mini sausage frittatas are perfectly portioned for quick breakfasts on the go. Make up a batch on the weekend and store them in the refrigerator or freezer for those hectic weekday mornings. They're also great to pack in a lunchbox or to take on a picnic. Make sure you read the label carefully and buy gluten-free sausage, or make your own (see the Chicken and Roasted Red Bell Pepper Sausage Patties recipe, page 67, and the Chicken-Apple Sausage Patties recipe, page 68).

NONSTICK COOKING SPRAY

8 OUNCES CRUMBLED
    BREAKFAST SAUSAGE

½ CUP FINELY DICED YELLOW ONION

SALT

FRESHLY GROUND BLACK PEPPER

5 EGGS

3 EGG WHITES

1 CUP FAT-FREE MILK

½ CUP SHREDDED CHEDDAR CHEESE

1. Preheat the oven to 325°F.

2. Spray 12 cups of a standard muffin tin with nonstick cooking spray.

3. In a medium skillet over medium-high heat, cook the sausage, stirring frequently and breaking up the chunks, until browned, about 3 minutes. With a slotted spoon, remove the sausage to a medium bowl and set aside.

4. Stir the onion into the sausage fat in the skillet, season with salt and pepper, and cook, stirring frequently, for 2 minutes. Spoon the onion into the bowl with the sausage.

5. In a medium bowl, whisk together the eggs, egg whites, and milk until well combined. Pour the egg mixture into the prepared muffin cups, dividing it evenly among the 12 cups.

6. Spoon 1 heaping tablespoon of the sausage-and-onion mixture into each cup. Top each cup with the shredded Cheddar cheese, evenly divided.

7. Bake the mini frittatas for 20 minutes, or until the eggs are puffed and set. Cool the mini frittatas for 5 minutes before serving.

NUTRITIONAL INFORMATION PER FRITTATA: CALORIES 123 TOTAL FAT 8.8G SATURATED FAT 3.3G
TRANS FAT 0.0G **SODIUM** 233MG **TOTAL CARBOHYDRATES** 1.7G **SUGARS** 1.4G **PROTEIN** 8.8G

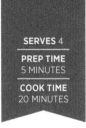
Sautéed Sweet Potatoes

No need to relegate sweet potatoes to a side dish at dinner. Their subtly sweet flavor and bright orange flesh make for a colorful breakfast that will brighten up your morning. Sweet potatoes are packed with vitamins C and D and beta-carotene to start you out right.

1 TABLESPOON EXTRA-VIRGIN
   OLIVE OIL

2 SWEET POTATOES, PEELED
   AND DICED

SALT

FRESHLY GROUND BLACK PEPPER

1 TEASPOON MINCED GARLIC

2 TABLESPOONS SLICED SCALLIONS

1. Heat the olive oil in a medium skillet over medium heat.

2. Add the sweet potatoes and toss to coat with oil. Season the sweet potatoes with salt and pepper.

3. Stir in the garlic and cook for 5 to 6 minutes, stirring often.

4. Sprinkle in the scallions and toss well. Cook for another 10 to 15 minutes, until the sweet potatoes are tender.

5. Spoon the sweet potatoes onto 4 plates and serve hot.

NUTRITIONAL INFORMATION PER SERVING: CALORIES 121 TOTAL FAT 3.6G SATURATED FAT 0.5G TRANS FAT 0.0G SODIUM 46MG TOTAL CARBOHYDRATES 21.4G SUGARS 0.0G PROTEIN 1.2G

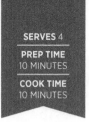
Easy Hash Browns

Crispy hash browns beat out toast any day as a side for scrambled eggs. This version is quick to prepare, and if you like your hash browns crispy and golden brown, it's definitely worth your time.

Cooking tip Wringing the moisture out of the potatoes is key to making these potatoes extra crispy. You could also try spinning them in a salad spinner to get the water out of them before frying.

3 TABLESPOONS EXTRA-VIRGIN
OLIVE OIL
1 POUND POTATOES, PEELED AND GRATED

SALT
FRESHLY GROUND BLACK PEPPER

1. Heat the olive oil in a large skillet over medium-high heat.

2. Spread the grated potatoes on a clean dish towel, then wrap and twist them, wringing as much moisture from them as possible.

3. Add the potatoes to the hot oil, spreading them in a thin layer. Season them with salt and pepper. Cook the potatoes in batches, if necessary, to keep the layer thin.

4. Cook until the underside of the potatoes is browned, about 3 minutes, then carefully flip them with a wide spatula and cook them until they are browned on the other side, about 3 minutes.

5. Transfer the potatoes to a warmed plate and repeat with any remaining potatoes.

6. Serve hot.

NUTRITIONAL INFORMATION PER SERVING: CALORIES 168 TOTAL FAT 10.6G SATURATED FAT 1.5G
TRANS FAT 0.0G SODIUM 46MG TOTAL CARBOHYDRATES 17.8G SUGARS 1.3G PROTEIN 1.9G

Chicken and Roasted Red Bell Pepper Sausage Patties

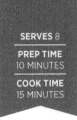

SERVES 8

PREP TIME
10 MINUTES

COOK TIME
15 MINUTES

Put down those store-bought sausage links. These homemade sausage patties are made with wholesome ingredients, packed with flavor, and so easy to make you won't believe it. You can substitute ground turkey or pork for the chicken, if you like.

1 TEASPOON EXTRA-VIRGIN OLIVE OIL

2 GARLIC CLOVES, MINCED

1 YELLOW ONION, DICED

1 POUND GROUND CHICKEN

¼ CUP CHOPPED ROASTED RED
    BELL PEPPER

1 TABLESPOON LIGHT BROWN SUGAR

½ TEASPOON SALT

¼ TEASPOON FRESHLY GROUND
    BLACK PEPPER

NONSTICK COOKING SPRAY

1. Heat the olive oil in a large skillet over medium heat.

2. Add the garlic and onion and cook for 2 minutes, until softened. Transfer the garlic and onion to a medium bowl.

3. In the same bowl, add the chicken, bell pepper, brown sugar, salt, and black pepper. Stir well to combine into a sausage mixture.

4. Spray the skillet with nonstick cooking spray and reheat it over medium heat.

5. Spoon the sausage mixture into the skillet using a ⅓-cup measure, making 4 patties at a time.

6. Gently flatten the 4 patties with a spatula and cook until they are browned on one side, about 5 minutes. Flip the patties and brown the other side, cooking for another 5 minutes.

7. Transfer the patties to a paper towel-lined plate to drain. Repeat the process with the remaining sausage mixture.

8. Serve hot.

NUTRITIONAL INFORMATION PER SERVING: CALORIES 126 TOTAL FAT 4.9G SATURATED FAT 1.2G
TRANS FAT 0.0G SODIUM 204MG TOTAL CARBOHYDRATES 2.9G SUGARS 1.8G PROTEIN 16.6G

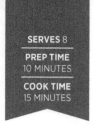

Chicken-Apple Sausage Patties

A little sweet, a little savory, and packed with protein, these sausage patties are just what you need to keep yourself full and focused throughout the morning. Go ahead and substitute any herbs you like—chives or thyme would be lovely—for the sage.

1 TEASPOON EXTRA-VIRGIN OLIVE OIL

1 GARLIC CLOVE, MINCED

1 YELLOW ONION, FINELY DICED

1 GREEN APPLE, PEELED, CORED, AND FINELY DICED

1 POUND GROUND CHICKEN

1 TABLESPOON LIGHT BROWN SUGAR

1 TABLESPOON CHOPPED FRESH SAGE

½ TEASPOON SALT

¼ TEASPOON FRESHLY GROUND BLACK PEPPER

NONSTICK COOKING SPRAY

1. Heat the olive oil in a large skillet over medium heat.

2. Add the garlic and onion and cook for 2 minutes, until softened.

3. Stir in the apple and cook for 2 minutes more, then transfer the mixture to a medium bowl.

4. In the same bowl, add the chicken, brown sugar, sage, salt, and pepper. Stir well to combine.

5. Spray the skillet with nonstick cooking spray and reheat it over medium heat.

6. Spoon the sausage mixture into the skillet using a ⅓-cup measure, making 4 patties at a time.

7. Gently flatten each patty with a spatula and cook until they are browned on one side, about 5 minutes. Flip the patties and brown the other side, about 5 minutes.

8. Transfer the patties to a paper towel-lined plate to drain. Repeat the process with the remaining sausage mixture. Serve hot.

NUTRITIONAL INFORMATION PER SERVING: CALORIES 137 TOTAL FAT 4.9G SATURATED FAT 1.3G TRANS FAT 0.0G SODIUM 197MG TOTAL CARBOHYDRATES 5.9G SUGARS 4.1G PROTEIN 16.6G

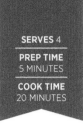

Peanut Butter Pancakes

In this recipe, brown rice flour produces hearty but tender pancakes loaded with peanut butter flavor. Top them with bananas and a drizzle of honey for a breakfast that's sure to keep you happy until lunch. For a more delicate version, substitute gluten-free all-purpose flour (homemade recipe on page 32) for the brown rice flour.

½ CUP BROWN RICE FLOUR
½ TEASPOON BAKING SODA
PINCH SALT
1 EGG
½ CUP PLAIN NONFAT YOGURT

1 TABLESPOON SMOOTH
PEANUT BUTTER
1 TEASPOON PURE MAPLE SYRUP
NONSTICK COOKING SPRAY

1. In a medium bowl, stir together the rice flour, baking soda, and salt.

2. In a separate medium bowl, beat together the egg, yogurt, peanut butter, and maple syrup.

3. Add the flour mixture to the egg mixture and whisk until well combined. The batter should be thick.

4. Spray a large skillet with nonstick cooking spray and heat it over medium heat.

5. Spoon the batter into the skillet, 2 to 3 tablespoons at a time, fitting as many pancakes as you can without overlapping. Cook the pancakes in batches so you don't crowd the skillet.

6. Let the pancakes cook for 2 minutes, or until they are golden brown underneath. Flip the pancakes and cook them until they are browned on the other side, about 2 minutes.

7. Transfer the pancakes to a warmed plate and repeat with the remaining batter.

8. Serve hot.

NUTRITIONAL INFORMATION PER SERVING: CALORIES 138   TOTAL FAT 4.2G   SATURATED FAT 1.2G
TRANS FAT 0.0G   **SODIUM** 237MG   **TOTAL CARBOHYDRATES** 19.2G   **SUGARS** 3.8G   **PROTEIN** 5.5G

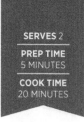

Three-Ingredient Banana Pancakes

It's hard to believe that a breakfast this delicious and nutritious can be made with just three ingredients. Quick and simple enough to prepare on a weekday morning, these pancakes are also vegan, dairy-free, grain-free, and kid-friendly. Serve them drizzled with honey or maple syrup.

2 BANANAS, PEELED AND CHOPPED

1 EGG, LIGHTLY BEATEN

1½ TABLESPOONS CASHEW BUTTER OR ALMOND BUTTER

NONSTICK COOKING SPRAY

1. Place the bananas in a medium bowl and mash them with a potato masher.

2. Stir in the egg and nut butter and mix until smooth.

3. Spray a skillet with nonstick cooking spray and heat it over medium heat.

4. Spoon the batter onto the skillet ¼ cup at a time, fitting as many pancakes as you can without overlapping. Cook the pancakes in batches so you don't crowd the skillet.

5. Let the pancakes cook for 2 minutes, or until they are golden brown underneath. Flip the pancakes and cook them until they are browned on the other side, about 2 minutes.

6. Transfer the pancakes to a warmed plate and repeat with the remaining batter.

7. Serve hot.

NUTRITIONAL INFORMATION PER SERVING: CALORIES 215   TOTAL FAT 9.2G   SATURATED FAT 1.5G
TRANS FAT 0.0G   SODIUM 32MG   TOTAL CARBOHYDRATES 29.2G   SUGARS 14.2G   PROTEIN 6.5G

Almond Flour Blueberry Pancakes

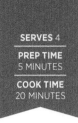

SERVES 4

PREP TIME
5 MINUTES

COOK TIME
20 MINUTES

Almond flour can be used to make many of your favorite recipes, including these blueberry pancakes. Almonds are full of omega-3 fatty acids, and blueberries are packed with antioxidants, making these tasty pancakes a true super food. Serve them drizzled with a bit of honey or maple syrup, if desired.

Ingredient tip If you don't have fresh blueberries, substitute frozen. And don't worry—you don't even need to thaw them before adding them to the pancakes.

1½ CUPS ALMOND FLOUR

3 EGGS

1 CUP FAT-FREE MILK

1 TEASPOON GROUND CINNAMON

PINCH SALT

NONSTICK COOKING SPRAY

1 CUP FRESH BLUEBERRIES

1. In a food processor or blender, combine the flour, eggs, milk, cinnamon, and salt, and blend until smooth.

2. Spray a large skillet with nonstick cooking spray and heat it over medium heat.

3. Spoon the batter onto the skillet, 2 to 3 tablespoons at a time, fitting as many pancakes as you can without overlapping.

4. Sprinkle a handful of the blueberries into the wet batter of each pancake. Cook the pancakes in batches so you don't crowd the skillet.

5. Let the pancakes cook for 2 minutes, or until they are golden brown underneath. Flip the pancakes and cook them until they are browned on the other side, about 2 minutes.

6. Transfer the pancakes to a warmed plate and repeat with the remaining batter.

7. Serve hot.

NUTRITIONAL INFORMATION PER SERVING: CALORIES 153 TOTAL FAT 8.8G SATURATED FAT 1.4G
TRANS FAT 0.0G SODIUM 122MG TOTAL CARBOHYDRATES 11.2G SUGARS 7.2G PROTEIN 8.7G

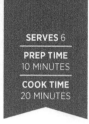
Pumpkin-Cinnamon Pancakes

Using coconut flour in this recipe makes these pancakes grain-free. Because coconut flour is lower in carbs than grain-based flours and higher in fiber than nut flours, these pancakes are a good choice if you are watching your weight. The addition of whey protein powder (look for it in health food stores) makes them a high-protein breakfast option for you and your family.

½ CUP COCONUT FLOUR

¼ CUP WHEY PROTEIN POWDER

1 TEASPOON BAKING POWDER

1 TEASPOON GROUND CINNAMON

½ TEASPOON SALT

¼ CUP PURE MAPLE SYRUP

6 EGGS

½ CUP PUMPKIN PURÉE

3 TABLESPOONS UNSALTED BUTTER,
    AT ROOM TEMPERATURE

½ CUP FAT-FREE MILK, PLUS MORE
    IF NEEDED

½ TEASPOON VANILLA EXTRACT

NONSTICK COOKING SPRAY

1. In a large bowl, combine the coconut flour, protein powder, baking powder, cinnamon, and salt.

2. In a medium bowl, whisk together the maple syrup, eggs, pumpkin, butter, milk, and vanilla.

3. Gradually beat the egg mixture into the flour mixture until it is just incorporated. Add more milk if needed to produce a thick batter.

4. Spray a large skillet with cooking spray and heat it over medium heat.

5. Spoon the batter onto the skillet, 2 tablespoons at a time, fitting as many pancakes as you can without overlapping. Cook the pancakes in batches so you don't crowd the skillet.

6. Let the pancakes cook for 2 minutes, or until they are golden brown underneath. Flip the pancakes and cook them until they are browned on the other side, about 2 minutes.

7. Transfer the pancakes to a warmed plate and repeat with the remaining batter.

NUTRITIONAL INFORMATION PER SERVING: CALORIES 227   TOTAL FAT 11.7G   SATURATED FAT 5.5G   TRANS FAT 0.0G
SODIUM 350MG   TOTAL CARBOHYDRATES 18.4G   DIETARY FIBER 4.4G   SUGARS 11.0G   PROTEIN 11.5G

Honey Drop Biscuits

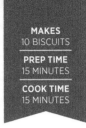

MAKES
10 BISCUITS

PREP TIME
15 MINUTES

COOK TIME
15 MINUTES

There's nothing quite like the aroma of buttery biscuits in the morning. Enjoy these little beauties smothered in homemade sausage gravy, stuffed with bacon and scrambled eggs, or spread with butter and your favorite fruit jam. You can also use this dough as a crispy topping for a cheesy sausage and egg casserole.

2½ CUPS ALMOND FLOUR, PLUS MORE FOR DUSTING

½ TEASPOON BAKING SODA

½ TEASPOON SALT

¼ CUP UNSALTED BUTTER, AT ROOM TEMPERATURE

2 EGGS

1½ TABLESPOONS HONEY

1. Preheat the oven to 350°F.

2. Line a baking sheet with parchment paper.

3. In a medium bowl, stir together the almond flour, baking soda, and salt.

4. In a separate medium bowl, whisk together the butter, eggs, and honey.

5. Stir the flour mixture into the egg mixture in small batches until just combined.

6. Roll out the dough on a floured work surface to about 1½ inches thick. Use the rim of a juice glass or a biscuit cutter to cut out 3-inch biscuits.

7. Place the biscuits on the prepared baking sheet, spacing them 1 inch apart.

8. Bake the biscuits for 15 minutes, until they are lightly browned. Allow them to cool slightly before serving.

NUTRITIONAL INFORMATION PER SERVING: **CALORIES** 103 **TOTAL FAT** 9.0G **SATURATED FAT** 3.4G **TRANS FAT** 0.0G **SODIUM** 227MG **TOTAL CARBOHYDRATES** 4.2G **SUGARS** 2.9G **PROTEIN** 2.7G

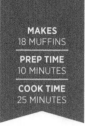

MAKES
18 MUFFINS

PREP TIME
10 MINUTES

COOK TIME
25 MINUTES

Carrot-Banana Muffins

These muffins are loaded with healthy ingredients: almond flour, bananas, honey, and carrots. Their sweet and nutty flavor makes them irresistible. Even the pickiest kids won't be able to resist eating their vegetables in these muffins.

Time-saving tip Bake a double batch. You can store leftover muffins in an airtight container at room temperature for up to 2 days, in the refrigerator for 2 to 4 days, and in the freezer for 2 to 4 months.

NONSTICK COOKING SPRAY

2 CUPS ALMOND FLOUR

2 TEASPOONS BAKING SODA

1 TEASPOON SALT

2 TEASPOONS GROUND CINNAMON

½ TEASPOON GROUND NUTMEG

½ CUP HONEY

3 BANANAS, CHOPPED

3 EGGS

1 TEASPOON APPLE CIDER VINEGAR

¼ CUP UNSALTED BUTTER, AT ROOM
   TEMPERATURE

1½ CUPS GRATED CARROTS

1. Preheat the oven to 350°F.

2. Spray 18 cups of 2 standard muffin tins with nonstick cooking spray.

3. In a medium bowl, combine the flour, baking soda, salt, cinnamon, and nutmeg.

4. In the bowl of a food processor or blender, combine the honey, bananas, eggs, vinegar, and butter. Blend until smooth.

5. Transfer the honey mixture to a large bowl and stir in the flour mixture in small batches until just combined. Fold in the carrots.

6. Spoon the batter into the muffin cups, filling each about two-thirds full.

7. Bake the muffins for 20 to 25 minutes, until they are lightly browned and cooked through (a toothpick inserted in the center of a muffin should come out clean).

8. Allow the muffins to cool for 5 minutes in the pan, then turn them out onto a wire rack to cool completely.

NUTRITIONAL INFORMATION PER SERVING: CALORIES 102 TOTAL FAT 4.9 SATURATED FAT 2.0G
TRANS FAT 0.0G SODIUM 304MG TOTAL CARBOHYDRATES 14.1G SUGARS 10.7G PROTEIN 1.9G

Raisin-Applesauce Muffins

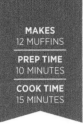

MAKES
12 MUFFINS

PREP TIME
10 MINUTES

COOK TIME
15 MINUTES

Coconut flour, which is loaded with fiber, is a very absorbent gluten-free flour, so you don't need much of it to make an entire batch of muffins. The applesauce, lots of eggs, and the addition of juicy raisins keep the muffins moist. You could even add a peeled, diced apple for even more apple flavor and a bit more moisture.

NONSTICK COOKING SPRAY

½ CUP COCONUT FLOUR

1 CUP UNSWEETENED APPLESAUCE

5 EGGS

¼ CUP COCONUT OIL

2 TABLESPOONS HONEY

2 TABLESPOONS GROUND CINNAMON

1 TEASPOON BAKING SODA

1 TEASPOON VANILLA EXTRACT

¼ TEASPOON SALT

½ CUP RAISINS

1. Preheat the oven to 400°F.

2. Spray 12 cups of a standard muffin pan with nonstick cooking spray.

3. In a food processor or blender, combine the flour, applesauce, eggs, coconut oil, honey, cinnamon, baking soda, vanilla, and salt, and blend until combined and smooth. Stir in the raisins.

4. Let the batter sit for 5 minutes, then spoon it into the muffin pan, filling each cup about two-thirds full.

5. Bake the muffins for 12 to 15 minutes, until the muffins are lightly browned and cooked through (a toothpick inserted in the center of a muffin should come out clean).

6. Allow the muffins to cool for 5 minutes in the pan, then turn them out onto a wire rack to cool completely.

7. Store leftover muffins in an airtight container at room temperature for up to 2 days, in the refrigerator for 2 to 4 days, and in the freezer for 2 to 4 months.

NUTRITIONAL INFORMATION PER SERVING: CALORIES 128   TOTAL FAT 7.0G   SATURATED FAT 4.7G
TRANS FAT 0.0G   **SODIUM** 191MG   **TOTAL CARBOHYDRATES** 13.7G   **SUGARS** 9.0G   **PROTEIN** 3.3G

MAKES
24 MINI MUFFINS

PREP TIME
10 MINUTES

COOK TIME
15 MINUTES

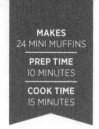

Chocolate Chip Mini Muffins

If you like to start your morning off with a little something sweet, give these muffins a try. They're made with almond flour, which provides the protein you need to keep you going, but the fact that they're studded with chocolate chips will make you smile.

2 CUPS ALMOND FLOUR

1 TEASPOON BAKING SODA

½ TEASPOON SALT

½ CUP UNSALTED BUTTER, AT ROOM
  TEMPERATURE

3 EGGS

½ CUP HONEY

¾ CUP MINI CHOCOLATE CHIPS

1. Preheat the oven to 350°F.

2. Line 24 cups of mini muffin pans with mini paper liners.

3. In a medium bowl, combine the flour, baking soda, and salt.

4. In a separate medium bowl, whisk together the butter, eggs, and honey.

5. Stir the egg mixture into the flour mixture until just combined. Fold in the chocolate chips.

6. Spoon the batter into the muffin cups, filling each one almost to the top.

7. Bake the muffins for 15 minutes, until they are cooked through. A toothpick inserted in the center of a muffin should come out clean.

8. Allow the muffins to cool in the pan for 5 minutes, then turn them out onto a wire rack to cool completely.

9. Store leftover muffins in an airtight container at room temperature for up to 2 days, in the refrigerator for 2 to 4 days, or in the freezer for 2 to 4 months.

NUTRITIONAL INFORMATION PER SERVING: **CALORIES** 81   **TOTAL FAT** 5.8G   **SATURATED FAT** 2.8G
TRANS FAT 0.0G   **SODIUM** 142MG   **TOTAL CARBOHYDRATES** 7.0G   **SUGARS** 6.2G   **PROTEIN** 1.3G

Lemon-Blueberry Mini Muffins

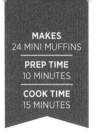

MAKES
24 MINI MUFFINS

PREP TIME
10 MINUTES

COOK TIME
15 MINUTES

These rich and sweet muffins taste like fancy little tea cakes. Made with almond flour, sweetened with honey, brightened with both lemon zest and lemon juice, and studded with fresh blueberries, they are just perfect for an on-the-go breakfast or a quick morning snack.

2 CUPS ALMOND FLOUR

1 TEASPOON BAKING SODA

½ TEASPOON SALT

½ CUP UNSALTED BUTTER, AT ROOM
 TEMPERATURE

3 EGGS

½ CUP HONEY

2 TABLESPOONS FRESHLY SQUEEZED
 LEMON JUICE

1 TEASPOON LEMON ZEST

1 CUP FRESH BLUEBERRIES

1. Preheat the oven to 350°F.

2. Line 24 cups of mini muffin pans with mini paper liners.

3. In a large bowl, combine the flour, baking soda, and salt.

4. In a medium bowl, whisk together the butter, eggs, honey, lemon juice, and lemon zest.

5. Stir the egg mixture into the flour mixture until just combined. Fold in the blueberries.

6. Spoon the batter into the muffin cups, filling each one almost to the top.

7. Bake the muffins for 15 minutes, until they are cooked through. A toothpick inserted in the center should come out clean.

8. Allow the muffins to cool in the pan for 5 minutes, then turn them out onto a wire rack to cool completely.

9. Store leftover muffins in an airtight container at room temperature for up to 2 days, in the refrigerator for 2 to 4 days, or in the freezer for 2 to 4 months.

NUTRITIONAL INFORMATION PER SERVING: CALORIES 80 TOTAL FAT 5.6G SATURATED FAT 2.7G
TRANS FAT 0.0G SODIUM 139MG TOTAL CARBOHYDRATES 7.3G SUGARS 6.5G PROTEIN 1.3G

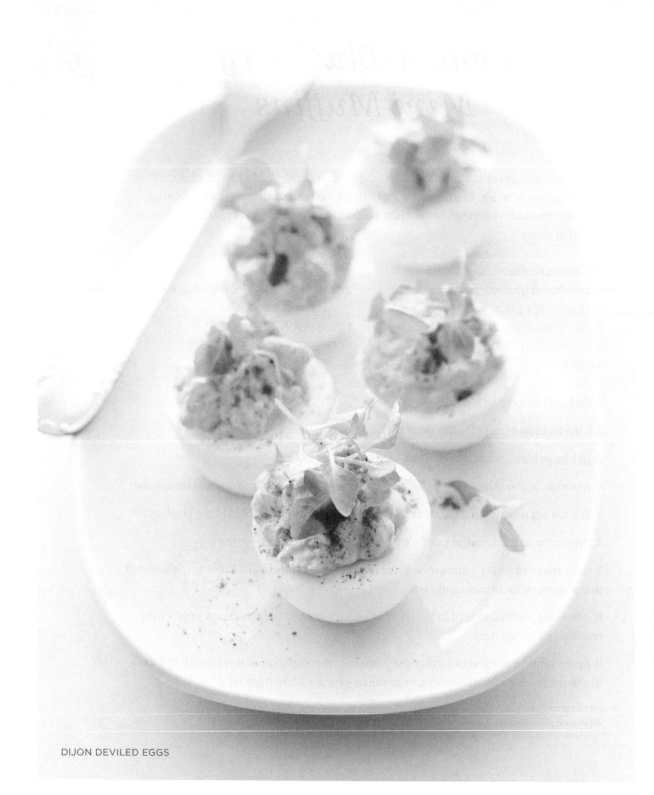

DIJON DEVILED EGGS

6

Appetizers and Snacks

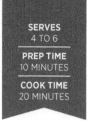

SERVES
4 TO 6

PREP TIME
10 MINUTES

COOK TIME
20 MINUTES

Easy Cinnamon Applesauce

Homemade applesauce is super easy to make. It's delicious on its own as a snack, or you can use it to top potato pancakes, oatmeal (gluten-free, of course!), or pork chops. Spoon it over ice cream, warm or cold. You can use it as a substitute for some or all of the fat in many baked goods, too.

Time-saving tip Cutting the apples into very small pieces reduces the cooking time. To reduce your prep time, you could cut the peeled, cored apples into quarters and pulse them into small pieces in a food processor.

4 GRANNY SMITH APPLES, PEELED, CORED, AND FINELY DICED

4 GOLDEN DELICIOUS APPLES, PEELED, CORED, AND FINELY DICED

¼ CUP UNSWEETENED APPLE JUICE

½ TEASPOON GROUND CINNAMON

PINCH GROUND NUTMEG

2 TO 4 TABLESPOONS SUGAR (OPTIONAL)

1. In a stockpot or Dutch oven over medium heat, combine the apples, apple juice, cinnamon, nutmeg, and sugar (if using).

2. Bring the mixture to a simmer. Stir occasionally and keep the sauce at a lively simmer for about 20 minutes, until the apples are very soft.

3. Transfer the mixture to a food processor or blender and process until smooth.

4. Serve immediately or store the applesauce in the refrigerator for up to 1 week.

NUTRITIONAL INFORMATION PER SERVING: CALORIES 220   TOTAL FAT 0.1G   TRANS FAT 0.0G
SODIUM 4MG   TOTAL CARBOHYDRATES 58.4G   SUGARS 45.6G   PROTEIN 0.0G

Lemon-Sesame Hummus

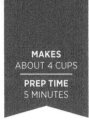

MAKES
ABOUT 4 CUPS

PREP TIME
5 MINUTES

Sure you can buy perfectly acceptable hummus at the supermarket, but this tangy, nutty lemon-sesame version is so bright and full of flavor that it's worth the minimal effort to make it yourself. Take a break from plain grocery store hummus and give this homemade version a try. You will be so pleased you did.

2 (15-OUNCE) CANS CHICKPEAS, DRAINED AND RINSED

¼ CUP FRESHLY SQUEEZED LEMON JUICE

1 GARLIC CLOVE, MINCED

¼ CUP SESAME SEEDS

¼ CUP WATER

SALT

1. In a food processor or blender, combine the chickpeas, lemon juice, garlic, and sesame seeds. Blend until smooth.

2. Add about half of the water and blend until smooth. Add more water, if needed, to thin the mixture.

3. Season the hummus with salt and chill until ready to serve.

4. The hummus can be stored in a sealed container in the refrigerator for 3 to 4 days.

NUTRITIONAL INFORMATION PER ½ CUP: **CALORIES** 415 **TOTAL FAT** 8.7G **SATURATED FAT** 1.0G **TRANS FAT** 0.0G **SODIUM** 47MG **TOTAL CARBOHYDRATES** 65.8G **SUGARS** 11.6G **PROTEIN** 21.4G

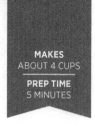

Roasted Red Pepper and Garlic Hummus

Using canned chickpeas and roasted red bell peppers and tahini (sesame seed paste) from a jar makes quick work of this flavorful hummus. Serve it alongside warm homemade Pita Bread (page 42) and fresh vegetable sticks for dipping, and this fresh, garlicky hummus will disappear before your eyes.

2 (15-OUNCE) CANS CHICKPEAS, DRAINED AND RINSED

¼ CUP ROASTED RED BELL PEPPER, CHOPPED

2 TABLESPOONS FRESHLY SQUEEZED LEMON JUICE

2 TABLESPOONS TAHINI

3 GARLIC CLOVES, MINCED

¼ CUP WATER, PLUS MORE IF NEEDED

SALT

1. In a food processor, combine the chickpeas, bell pepper, lemon juice, tahini, and garlic. Blend until smooth.

2. Add about half of the water and blend until smooth. Add more water, if needed, to thin the mixture.

3. Season the hummus with salt and chill until ready to serve.

4. This hummus can be stored in the refrigerator in a sealed container for 3 to 4 days.

NUTRITIONAL INFORMATION PER ½ CUP: CALORIES 414 TOTAL FAT 8.5G SATURATED FAT 1.0G TRANS FAT 0.0G SODIUM 65MG TOTAL CARBOHYDRATES 66.2G SUGARS 11.7G PROTEIN 21.3G

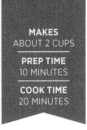

MAKES
ABOUT 2 CUPS

PREP TIME
10 MINUTES

COOK TIME
20 MINUTES

Spicy Artichoke Dip

A spicy twist on a classic dish, this artichoke dip is sure to surprise and guaranteed to please. It's enriched with nutty tahini and rich sour cream and gets a kick from cayenne pepper. Serve it with warm homemade Pita Bread (page 42) or homemade Multigrain Crackers (page 90) for an award-worthy spread.

1 (12-OUNCE) PACKAGE FROZEN
    ARTICHOKE HEARTS, THAWED
1 GARLIC CLOVE, PEELED
1 TABLESPOON MINCED RED ONION
½ CUP TAHINI
½ CUP SOUR CREAM
1 TABLESPOON FRESHLY GRATED
    PARMESAN CHEESE

1 TABLESPOON FRESHLY SQUEEZED
    LEMON JUICE
SALT
FRESHLY GROUND BLACK PEPPER
¼ TEASPOON CAYENNE PEPPER
1 TEASPOON UNSALTED BUTTER
3 TABLESPOONS SLICED ALMONDS

1. Preheat the oven to 375°F.

2. In a food processor or blender, combine the artichoke hearts and garlic and pulse until finely chopped.

3. Spoon the mixture into a medium bowl and stir in the onion, tahini, sour cream, Parmesan cheese, and lemon juice. Season the mixture with salt and black pepper and stir in the cayenne.

4. Spoon the mixture into a small baking dish and set aside.

5. In a small skillet over medium-low heat, melt the butter. Add the almonds and stir well. Toast the almonds for 2 to 3 minutes, until lightly browned.

6. Sprinkle the almonds over the artichoke dip.

7. Bake the dip for 15 minutes, or until hot and bubbling. Serve immediately.

NUTRITIONAL INFORMATION PER ½ CUP: CALORIES 340   TOTAL FAT 27.0G   SATURATED FAT 7.8G
TRANS FAT 0.0G   SODIUM 241MG   TOTAL CARBOHYDRATES 18.4G   SUGARS 1.4G   PROTEIN 12.1G

MAKES
4 TO 5 CUPS

PREP TIME
10 MINUTES

COOK TIME
25 MINUTES

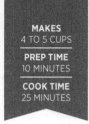

Spinach-Onion Dip

With bacon, sour cream, cream cheese, and spinach, this gluten-free recipe maintains all the delicious flavor of the classic dish. Serve it with homemade Multigrain Crackers (page 90) or gluten-free French bread and fresh vegetable sticks for dipping.

4 SLICES BACON, CHOPPED

1 YELLOW ONION, DICED

SALT

FRESHLY GROUND BLACK PEPPER

1 TEASPOON COCONUT FLOUR

2 (10-OUNCE) PACKAGES FROZEN
   SPINACH, THAWED AND DRAINED

1 CUP WHOLE MILK

½ CUP LIGHT SOUR CREAM

8 OUNCES CREAM CHEESE, AT ROOM
   TEMPERATURE

6 TABLESPOONS FRESHLY GRATED
   PARMESAN CHEESE

1. Preheat the oven to 350°F.

2. In a medium skillet over medium-high heat, cook the bacon, stirring often, for 4 minutes, or until crisp. Use a slotted spoon to transfer the bacon to a paper towel-lined plate to drain.

3. Remove all but about 2 teaspoons of bacon fat from the skillet and reheat it over medium heat.

4. Add the onion and season it with salt and pepper. Cook for 5 minutes while stirring.

5. Stir in the coconut flour and cook, stirring, for 30 seconds.

6. Add the spinach, milk, sour cream, and cream cheese, and stir to combine well. Cook for 2 minutes, stirring frequently, until the mixture melts. Stir in the bacon and 3 tablespoons of Parmesan cheese.

7. Spoon the mixture into a medium baking dish and top with the remaining 3 tablespoons of Parmesan cheese.

8. Bake the dip for 15 minutes, until it's hot and bubbling. Let it sit for 5 minutes before serving hot.

NUTRITIONAL INFORMATION PER ½ CUP: CALORIES 268   TOTAL FAT 21.2G   SATURATED FAT 12.0G
TRANS FAT 0.0G   SODIUM 529MG   TOTAL CARBOHYDRATES 7.4G   SUGARS 2.6G   PROTEIN 13.8G

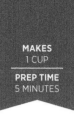

Homemade Basil Pesto

Enjoy this homemade basil pesto on hot gluten-free toast, topped with a dollop of tangy goat cheese, for a filling appetizer. Or stir it into your favorite gluten-free pasta, along with chopped roasted chicken and steamed or roasted broccoli, for a tasty meal.

Time-saving tip Pesto freezes well and is a great quick and easy way to add flavor to soups and sauces. Make a large batch and freeze the extra in an ice cube tray. Transfer the frozen cubes to a resealable plastic bag. Any time you want a bit of fresh, herby flavor in a dish or need a quick pasta sauce, pull out as many cubes as you need.

2 CUPS GENTLY PACKED FRESH BASIL

⅓ CUP WALNUTS

½ CUP FRESHLY GRATED
    ROMANO CHEESE

1 TEASPOON MINCED GARLIC

½ CUP EXTRA-VIRGIN OLIVE OIL

SALT

FRESHLY GROUND BLACK PEPPER

1. In a food processor or blender, combine the basil and walnuts and pulse until they are finely chopped.

2. Add the Romano cheese and garlic and pulse several more times to combine.

3. With the food processor running, drizzle in the olive oil in a slow, steady stream.

4. Season the pesto with salt and pepper.

5. The pesto can be stored in an airtight container in the refrigerator for up to 1 week and in the freezer for up to 6 months.

NUTRITIONAL INFORMATION PER 2 TABLESPOONS: CALORIES 227 TOTAL FAT 22.0G SATURATED FAT 5.1G
TRANS FAT 0.0G SODIUM 233MG TOTAL CARBOHYDRATES 1.7G SUGAR 0.0G PROTEIN 7.7G

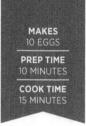

MAKES
10 EGGS

PREP TIME
10 MINUTES

COOK TIME
15 MINUTES

Dijon Deviled Eggs

Deviled eggs are a classic party dish, and this old-school version, spiked with Dijon mustard, won't disappoint. You could add any number of additional ingredients—minced anchovies, minced chiles, chopped capers, minced chives, minced kalamata olives, or sriracha sauce—for variety.

Cooking tip Use a pastry bag to pipe the filling into the egg white halves for a simple but professional-looking presentation. If you don't have a reusable pastry bag, inexpensive disposable pastry bags are available at most supermarkets. Or you can make your own by snipping the corner off a heavy-duty zip-top bag.

5 HARDBOILED EGGS, COOLED AND PEELED

1½ TABLESPOONS MAYONNAISE

1 TABLESPOON DIJON MUSTARD

3 TABLESPOONS FINELY DICED CELERY

1 TABLESPOON MINCED WHITE ONION

3 TABLESPOONS MINCED FRESH FLAT-LEAF PARSLEY

SALT

FRESHLY GROUND BLACK PEPPER

1. Cut the hardboiled eggs in half lengthwise.

2. Scoop the yolks into a small bowl. Arrange the egg whites on a serving dish.

3. Mash the egg yolks with a fork and stir in the mayonnaise, Dijon mustard, celery, onion, and parsley. Season the mixture with salt and pepper.

4. Spoon or pipe the egg yolk filling into the egg white halves.

5. Cover and chill the eggs until ready to serve.

NUTRITIONAL INFORMATION PER ½ EGG: CALORIES 42 TOTAL FAT 3.0G SATURATED FAT 0.8G TRANS FAT 0.0G SODIUM 82MG TOTAL CARBOHYDRATES 1.0G SUGAR 0.0G PROTEIN 2.9G

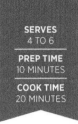

SERVES
4 TO 6

PREP TIME
10 MINUTES

COOK TIME
20 MINUTES

Goat Cheese and Herb-Stuffed Mushrooms

Stuff your mushrooms with a flavorful mixture of creamy goat cheese and fresh herbs, and you won't even miss the bread crumb topping. This recipe is so easy to prepare and so tasty that it may become your favorite party appetizer.

Cooking tip Mushrooms absorb a great deal of water. To keep them from getting mushy, gently wipe them clean with a paper towel; do not rinse them under running water or immerse them in a bowl of water.

1 POUND WHOLE WHITE BUTTON
    MUSHROOMS

8 OUNCES CRUMBLED GOAT CHEESE

1 TEASPOON MINCED GARLIC

3 TABLESPOONS CHOPPED FRESH FLAT-
    LEAF PARSLEY (LEAVES ONLY)

1 TABLESPOON CHOPPED
    FRESH CHIVES

1 TABLESPOON CHOPPED FRESH BASIL

SALT

FRESHLY GROUND BLACK PEPPER

1. Preheat the oven to 400°F.

2. Line a baking sheet with parchment paper.

3. Clean the mushrooms with a damp paper towel and remove the stems.

4. Arrange the mushrooms caps cup-side up on the prepared baking sheet.

5. In a food processor or blender, combine the goat cheese, garlic, parsley, chives, and basil, and blend until smooth. Or beat the mixture by hand in a large bowl.

6. Season the mixture with salt and pepper.

7. Spoon about 1 teaspoon of the mixture into each mushroom cap.

8. Bake the mushrooms for 20 minutes, or until the tops are lightly browned. Allow the mushrooms to cool slightly before serving warm.

NUTRITIONAL INFORMATION PER SERVING: CALORIES 285 TOTAL FAT 20.2G SATURATED FAT 13.9G
TRANS FAT 0.0G SODIUM 257MG TOTAL CARBOHYDRATES 5.7G SUGARS 1.3G PROTEIN 21.4G

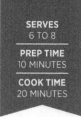

SERVES
6 TO 8

PREP TIME
10 MINUTES

COOK TIME
20 MINUTES

Smoky Prosciutto-Wrapped Squash

Butternut squash is a delicious, nutritious stand-in for the usual shrimp in this recipe. If you don't have prosciutto, substitute bacon. This is a great dish to serve in the fall and winter, when butternut squash is at its prime.

1 TABLESPOON EXTRA-VIRGIN
    OLIVE OIL

1 GARLIC CLOVE, MINCED

1 TEASPOON GROUND CHIPOTLE PEPPER

1 TEASPOON FRESHLY GROUND
    BLACK PEPPER

¼ TEASPOON SALT

½ SMALL BUTTERNUT SQUASH,
    PEELED, SEEDED, AND CUT
    INTO STICKS

8 OUNCES VERY THINLY SLICED
    PROSCIUTTO, CUT INTO STRIPS

1. Preheat the oven to 350°F.

2. In a large bowl, stir together the olive oil, garlic, chipotle pepper, black pepper, and salt. Add the squash sticks and toss to coat well.

3. Wrap a squash stick with a strip of prosciutto and lay it on a baking sheet. Repeat with the remaining squash and prosciutto.

4. Bake the squash for about 20 minutes, turning them once halfway through, until the prosciutto is crisp and the squash is tender. Serve hot.

NUTRITIONAL INFORMATION PER SERVING: CALORIES 135 TOTAL FAT 6.5G SATURATED FAT 1.7G
TRANS FAT 0.0G **SODIUM** 982MG **TOTAL CARBOHYDRATES** 10.2G **SUGARS** 1.6G **PROTEIN** 11.6G

Crisp Rosemary Crackers

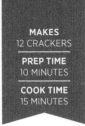

MAKES
12 CRACKERS

PREP TIME
10 MINUTES

COOK TIME
15 MINUTES

These rosemary crackers are a great crunchy snack. Not only is rosemary a flavorful and aromatic herb, but it also provides anti-inflammatory benefits. With only five ingredients, this recipe could not be any simpler.

1¾ CUPS ALMOND FLOUR

2 TABLESPOONS FINELY CHOPPED
    FRESH ROSEMARY LEAVES

½ TEASPOON SALT

1 EGG

1 TABLESPOON EXTRA-VIRGIN
    OLIVE OIL

1. In a medium bowl, add the almond flour, rosemary, and salt and stir to combine.

2. In a separate small bowl, whisk together the egg and olive oil.

3. Stir the egg mixture into the flour mixture in small batches until well combined.

4. Gather the dough into a ball and place it between 2 sheets of parchment paper. With a rolling pin, roll the dough out until it is about ⅛ inch thick.

5. Remove the parchment paper from the top of the dough. Using the bottom sheet, transfer the dough onto a baking sheet, still on the paper.

6. Use a pizza cutter to cut the dough into 2-inch squares.

7. Bake the crackers for 12 to 15 minutes, until they are golden and crisp.

8. Allow the crackers to cool on the baking sheet for 30 minutes before serving.

NUTRITIONAL INFORMATION PER SERVING: CALORIES 40   **TOTAL FAT** 3.6G   **TRANS FAT** 0.0G
SODIUM 104MG   **TOTAL CARBOHYDRATES** 1.2G   **SUGAR** 0.0G   **PROTEIN** 1.4G

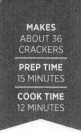

MAKES
ABOUT 36
CRACKERS

PREP TIME
15 MINUTES

COOK TIME
12 MINUTES

Multigrain Crackers

These crisp crackers are full of whole-grain goodness. Serve them alongside a cheese or charcuterie platter or as a dipper for dips like Lemon-Sesame Hummus (page 81) and Roasted Red Pepper and Garlic Hummus (page 82), Spinach-Onion Dip (page 84), or Spicy Artichoke Dip (page 83).

Ingredient tip Nutritional yeast is yeast that has been heated until the yeast is no longer active. As a result, it loses that yeasty flavor and actually tastes nutty and cheesy. In fact, many vegans use it as a cheese-flavoring substitute. Nutritional yeast is an excellent source of B vitamins and protein. It comes in powdered and flake form, and you can find it in health food stores and online.

½ CUP ALMOND FLOUR

¼ CUP SORGHUM FLOUR

¼ CUP TAPIOCA STARCH

2 TABLESPOONS TEFF FLOUR

2 TABLESPOONS NUTRITIONAL
   YEAST POWDER

2 TABLESPOONS GOLDEN
   FLAXSEED MEAL

2 TABLESPOONS MILLET FLOUR

¼ CUP UNSALTED BUTTER, AT ROOM
   TEMPERATURE

½ TEASPOON SALT, PLUS MORE FOR
   SPRINKLING

2 TO 4 TABLESPOONS WATER

1. Preheat the oven to 400°F.

2. Line a baking sheet with parchment paper.

3. In the bowl of a food processor, combine the almond flour, sorghum flour, tapioca starch, teff flour, nutritional yeast, flaxseed meal, millet flour, butter, and salt. Pulse to mix well. Or mix and beat the ingredients in a large bowl.

4. Add the water, 1 tablespoon at a time, and process for 30 seconds or so (or beat by hand) after each addition, until a cohesive dough forms. Continue adding water until the dough holds together, but not so much that it becomes sticky.

5. Lightly flour your work surface with any gluten-free flour. Turn the dough out onto the floured work surface and use a rolling pin to roll it out to an even thickness of about ¼ inch or thinner.

6. Use a pastry cutter or sharp knife to cut the dough into individual crackers. Set the crackers on the prepared baking sheet with at least ¼ inch of space between each cracker. Poke several holes in each cracker with the tines of a fork. Sprinkle the crackers with salt.

7. Bake the crackers for 10 to 12 minutes, until they are lightly browned. Transfer the crackers to a cooling rack and let them cool before serving.

8. Store extra crackers in an airtight container for 3 to 4 days, or pop them in the freezer to store them for up to 3 months.

NUTRITIONAL INFORMATION PER SERVING: CALORIES 28 TOTAL FAT 1.7G SATURATED FAT 0.8G
TRANS FAT 0.0G SODIUM 41MG TOTAL CARBOHYDRATES 2.8G SUGAR 0.0G PROTEIN 0.7G

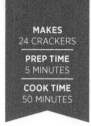

MAKES
24 CRACKERS

PREP TIME
5 MINUTES

COOK TIME
50 MINUTES

Chia Seed Crackers

These crunchy crackers have no grains, eggs, or dairy in them. What they do have is a whole lot of healthy fats, omega-3 fatty acids, protein, fiber, and minerals—and an amazing nutty flavor. They make a great snack on their own and are also great for dipping in homemade dips like Lemon-Sesame Hummus (page 81), Roasted Red Pepper and Garlic Hummus (page 82), Spinach-Onion Dip (page 84), or Spicy Artichoke Dip (page 83).

¾ CUP CHIA SEEDS

½ CUP PUMPKIN SEEDS

½ CUP SUNFLOWER SEEDS

¼ CUP SESAME SEEDS

1 CUP WATER

¼ TEASPOON KOSHER SALT

1. Preheat the oven to 325°F.

2. Line a baking sheet with parchment paper.

3. In a medium bowl, stir together the chia seeds, pumpkin seeds, sunflower seeds, sesame seeds, water, and salt until thick and well combined.

4. Spread the mixture on the prepared baking sheet about ¼ inch thick.

5. Bake the crackers for 30 minutes, then remove them from the oven. Use a pizza cutter to slice the crackers into 2-inch squares.

6. Flip the crackers carefully and bake them for another 20 to 25 minutes.

7. Allow the crackers to cool completely before serving.

NUTRITIONAL INFORMATION PER SERVING: CALORIES 44 TOTAL FAT 3.8G SATURATED FAT 0.0G
TRANS FAT 0.0G SODIUM 24MG TOTAL CARBOHYDRATES 2.5G SUGAR 0.0G PROTEIN 1.9G

Curried Almonds

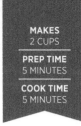
MAKES
2 CUPS

PREP TIME
5 MINUTES

COOK TIME
5 MINUTES

If you are looking for a healthy snack, try these curried nuts. Almonds are a rich source of omega-3 fatty acids and protein. Tossed in a spicy mix of curry and black pepper, they are perfectly addictive.

Ingredient tip Be sure to read the label on your curry powder because some mixtures contain wheat. If you can't find one that's wheat-free, make your own by combining 4 tablespoons of ground coriander, 2 tablespoons of ground turmeric, 2 tablespoons of dry mustard powder, 2 tablespoons of chili powder, 1 tablespoon of cayenne pepper, 1 tablespoon of ground cumin, and 1½ teaspoons of ground cardamom.

1 TABLESPOON CANOLA OIL

2 CUPS WHOLE RAW ALMONDS

1 TEASPOON GROUND TURMERIC

1 TEASPOON SALT

¼ TEASPOON CURRY POWDER

¼ TEASPOON FRESHLY GROUND
BLACK PEPPER

1. Heat the canola oil in a heavy medium skillet over medium heat.

2. Add the almonds and toss to coat. Stir in the turmeric, salt, curry powder, and pepper.

3. Toast the almonds, stirring occasionally, for about 5 minutes.

4. Remove the almonds from the heat and allow them to cool in the pan before serving.

5. Store the almonds in an airtight container in a cool, dry pantry cupboard for 2 to 4 months or in the refrigerator for up to 6 months.

NUTRITIONAL INFORMATION PER ½ CUP: CALORIES 124 TOTAL FAT 11.6G SATURATED FAT 1.0G TRANS FAT 0.0G SODIUM 582MG TOTAL CARBOHYDRATES 3.5G SUGARS 1.0G PROTEIN 3.1G

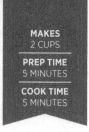

MAKES
2 CUPS

PREP TIME
5 MINUTES

COOK TIME
5 MINUTES

Roasted Vanilla Walnuts

Rich walnuts are flavored with intense vanilla bean and sweetened with a touch of honey for a delicately sweet but boldly flavored snack. If you don't have walnuts, you can substitute pecans, almonds, or even cashews. You might even try a mix of nuts.

1 TABLESPOON CANOLA OIL

2 CUPS WALNUT HALVES

2 TABLESPOONS HONEY

PINCH SALT

2 WHOLE VANILLA BEANS

1. Heat the canola oil in a heavy medium skillet over medium heat. Stir in the walnuts and toss to coat with oil.

2. Toast the walnuts for 3 to 5 minutes, until fragrant, then stir in the honey and salt.

3. Use a small, sharp knife to slice open the vanilla beans lengthwise. Scrape the seeds into the skillet. (Reserve the pods for another use, if desired.)

4. Stir the mixture well and remove the pan from the heat. Allow the walnuts to cool before serving.

5. Store the walnuts in an airtight container in the refrigerator for up to 1 month.

NUTRITIONAL INFORMATION PER 2 TABLESPOONS: CALORIES 225   TOTAL FAT 20.2G   SATURATED FAT 1.2G
TRANS FAT 0.0G   SODIUM 20MG   TOTAL CARBOHYDRATES 7.4G   SUGARS 4.6G   PROTEIN 7.5G

Honey-Glazed Pecans

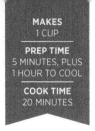

MAKES
1 CUP

PREP TIME
5 MINUTES, PLUS
1 HOUR TO COOL

COOK TIME
20 MINUTES

These honey-glazed pecans are a simple sweet treat that can be served as a snack or given away as a tasty holiday gift. You can substitute any unsalted nuts, or a mixture, for the pecans. Even peanuts will work in this recipe.

Time-saving tip You can make these nuts in big batches and store them in an airtight container in a cool, dry pantry cupboard for 2 to 4 weeks and in the refrigerator for up to 9 months.

⅓ CUP HONEY

1 TABLESPOON LIGHT BROWN SUGAR

1 CUP SHELLED PECAN HALVES

1. Preheat the oven to 350°F.

2. Line a baking sheet with foil.

3. In a small saucepan over medium heat, combine the honey and brown sugar and cook, stirring constantly, until the mixture is well combined and the sugar is dissolved, about 3 minutes.

4. Add the pecans to the honey mixture and toss to coat, then spread them out in a single layer on the prepared baking sheet.

5. Bake the pecans for 12 minutes, then stir, and bake them for an additional 3 to 5 minutes, until they are lightly toasted.

6. Allow the pecans to cool for 1 hour, then break the glazed nuts apart to serve.

NUTRITIONAL INFORMATION PER ¼ CUP: CALORIES 288 TOTAL FAT 20.0G SATURATED FAT 2.0G
TRANS FAT 0.0G SODIUM 2MG TOTAL CARBOHYDRATES 27.8G SUGARS 24.7G PROTEIN 3.1G

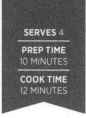

Crispy Coconut Shrimp

These crispy shrimp, flavored with rich coconut, make an elegant appetizer that your guests will love. Serve them as they are or with a Thai-style sweet chili sauce for dipping. In this recipe, use any type of gluten-free bread crumbs or bread crumb substitute that you like.

Time-saving tip Peeling and deveining shrimp is a time-consuming task. To save time, buy shrimp that's already been peeled and deveined. It costs a little more, but it's worth it.

1¼ POUNDS LARGE SHRIMP, PEELED AND DEVEINED, TAILS LEFT ON

½ CUP GLUTEN-FREE BREAD CRUMBS

¾ CUP UNSWEETENED FLAKED COCONUT

¾ TEASPOON GARLIC POWDER

¼ TEASPOON SALT

2 EGG WHITES, AT ROOM TEMPERATURE

1. Preheat the oven to 425°F.

2. Line 2 baking sheets with parchment paper.

3. Use a small, sharp knife to cut along the backs of the shrimp, butterflying them without cutting them in half.

4. In a shallow dish, stir together the bread crumbs, coconut, garlic powder, and salt.

5. In a separate shallow dish, beat the egg whites until foamy.

6. Toss the shrimp with the egg whites to coat, then dredge them in the coconut mixture.

7. Place the shrimp on the prepared baking sheet and bake them for 6 minutes.

8. Turn the shrimp and bake them for another 5 to 6 minutes, until the coating is crisp and browned.

9. Serve hot.

NUTRITIONAL INFORMATION PER SERVING: CALORIES 257 TOTAL FAT 7.7G SATURATED FAT 5.8G
TRANS FAT 0.0G SODIUM 442MG TOTAL CARBOHYDRATES 18.0G SUGARS 1.8G PROTEIN 30.3G

Baked Chicken Nuggets

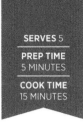

Going gluten-free can be especially tricky when your household includes small children, who are known for being particular about their favorite foods. These gluten-free chicken nuggets, though, are sure to please. It's an added bonus that they are baked in the oven instead of being fried, so they have less fat and fewer calories. Gluten-free baking mix—a combination of gluten-free flours and other ingredients such as xanthan or guar gum—is available in any health food or natural foods store and many supermarkets.

Time-saving tip Instead of buying whole chicken breasts and cutting them up, use boneless chicken breast tenders, which are already in small pieces.

¾ CUP GLUTEN-FREE BAKING MIX

½ CUP FRESHLY GRATED
    PARMESAN CHEESE

SALT

FRESHLY GROUND BLACK PEPPER

2 EGGS

1 POUND BONELESS SKINLESS
    CHICKEN BREAST, CUT INTO
    2-INCH CUBES

1. Preheat the oven to 450°F.

2. Line a baking sheet with parchment paper.

3. In a shallow dish, combine the baking mix and Parmesan cheese. Season the mixture with salt and pepper.

4. In a small bowl, beat the eggs. Dip the chicken cubes into the egg to coat them, then dredge the chicken in the baking mix.

5. Spread out the chicken cubes on the baking sheet and bake them for 12 to 15 minutes, turning once halfway through, until they are cooked through and golden brown.

NUTRITIONAL INFORMATION PER SERVING: CALORIES 328   **TOTAL FAT** 13.5G   **SATURATED FAT** 5.6G
TRANS FAT 0.0G   **SODIUM** 490MG   **TOTAL CARBOHYDRATES** 14.5G   **SUGAR** 0.0G   **PROTEIN** 36.6G

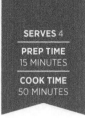

Spicy Buffalo Wings

When planning what to serve while you watch the big game, don't forget to include these spicy Buffalo wings, which are sure to score big points with guests. For a classic presentation, serve them with a gluten-free blue cheese dip and celery and carrot sticks.

2 POUNDS CHICKEN WINGS

3 TABLESPOONS HOT SAUCE

2 TABLESPOONS MELTED BUTTER

1 TEASPOON WORCESTERSHIRE SAUCE

PINCH CAYENNE PEPPER

1. Preheat the oven to 450°F.

2. Line a baking sheet with foil.

3. Heat a large pot of salted water over medium-high heat to boiling, then add the chicken wings. Boil the wings for 8 to 9 minutes, then drain them on a wire rack.

4. Transfer the wings to the prepared baking sheet and bake them for 25 minutes. Turn the wings over, then bake them for another 10 to 15 minutes, until they are cooked through. Remove the wings from the oven and place them in a large bowl.

5. In a medium saucepan over medium heat, cook the hot sauce, butter, Worcestershire, and cayenne until the butter is melted.

6. Whisk the sauce smooth, then add the cooked chicken wings and toss to coat.

7. Serve immediately.

NUTRITIONAL INFORMATION PER SERVING: CALORIES 484 TOTAL FAT 22.6G SATURATED FAT 8.3G TRANS FAT 0.0G SODIUM 535MG TOTAL CARBOHYDRATES 0.5G SUGAR 0.0G PROTEIN 65.7G

Honey-Barbecue Wings

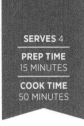

SERVES 4

PREP TIME
15 MINUTES

COOK TIME
50 MINUTES

If you prefer sweet to spicy, these barbecued wings will hit the spot. Coated with a finger-licking glaze of barbecue sauce and honey, they are as addictive as the best junk food, but, aside from a bit of sugar, perfectly healthy.

Ingredient tip If you're using a store-bought barbecue sauce, read the label carefully. Many commercial sauces contain gluten in the form of thickeners, emulsifiers, and natural flavors.

2 POUNDS CHICKEN WINGS

3 TABLESPOONS BARBECUE SAUCE

1 TABLESPOON MELTED BUTTER

1 TABLESPOON HONEY

1. Preheat the oven to 450°F.

2. Line a baking sheet with foil.

3. Heat a large pot of salted water over medium-high heat to boiling, then add the chicken wings. Boil the wings for 8 to 9 minutes, then drain them on a wire rack.

4. Transfer the wings to the prepared baking sheet and bake them for 25 minutes. Turn the wings over, then bake them for another 10 to 15 minutes, until they are cooked through. Remove the wings from the oven and place them in a large bowl.

5. In a medium saucepan over medium heat, cook the barbecue sauce, butter, and honey until the butter is melted.

6. Whisk the sauce smooth, then add the wings and toss to coat.

7. Serve immediately.

NUTRITIONAL INFORMATION PER SERVING: CALORIES 490 TOTAL FAT 19.7G SATURATED FAT 6.5G
TRANS FAT 0.0G SODIUM 347MG TOTAL CARBOHYDRATES 8.6G SUGARS 7.4G PROTEIN 65.7G

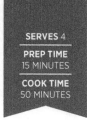

Maple and Soy Wings

The world can never have too many variations of sweet-salty chicken wings. This version is a tried-and-true favorite that's sure to be a winner at your house. Kids especially love these maple syrup-sweetened wings.

2 POUNDS CHICKEN WINGS

3 TABLESPOONS GLUTEN-FREE
    SOY SAUCE

1 TABLESPOON BUTTER

1 TABLESPOON PURE MAPLE SYRUP

2 TABLESPOONS SLICED SCALLIONS

1 TABLESPOON SESAME SEEDS

1. Preheat the oven to 450°F.

2. Line a baking sheet with foil.

3. Heat a large pot of salted water over medium-high heat to boiling, then add the chicken wings. Boil the wings for 8 to 9 minutes, then drain them on a wire rack.

4. Transfer the wings to the prepared baking sheet and bake them for 25 minutes. Turn the wings over, then bake them for another 10 to 15 minutes, until they are cooked through. Remove the wings from the oven and place them in a large bowl.

5. In a medium saucepan over medium heat, cook the soy sauce, butter, and maple syrup until the butter is melted. Add the scallions and sesame seeds.

6. Whisk the sauce smooth, then add the wings and toss to coat.

7. Serve immediately.

NUTRITIONAL INFORMATION PER SERVING: CALORIES 491 TOTAL FAT 20.8G SATURATED FAT 6.6G
TRANS FAT 0.0G **SODIUM** 952MG **TOTAL CARBOHYDRATES** 4.8G **SUGARS** 3.1G **PROTEIN** 67.6G

Mini Turkey Meatballs with Sweet-and-Sour Sauce

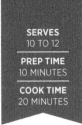

SERVES
10 TO 12

PREP TIME
10 MINUTES

COOK TIME
20 MINUTES

These sweet-and-sour meatballs are grain-free, made with naturally low-fat ground turkey, and sweetened only with pineapple and pineapple juice. They are sure to be a hit at your next cocktail party. Serve them on a platter with toothpicks for grabbing.

1⅓ POUNDS GROUND TURKEY

3 GARLIC CLOVES, MINCED

1 TABLESPOON MINCED FRESH GINGER

SALT

FRESHLY GROUND BLACK PEPPER

1 TABLESPOON COCONUT OIL

1 RED BELL PEPPER, CUT INTO
   1-INCH SQUARES

1 (20-OUNCE) CAN PINEAPPLE
   CHUNKS, IN JUICE

1 TABLESPOON ARROWROOT STARCH

1 BUNCH SCALLIONS, THINLY SLICED,
   FOR GARNISH

1. Preheat the oven to 400°F.

2. In a medium bowl, combine the ground turkey, garlic, and ginger, and mix well. Season the mixture with salt and black pepper.

3. Form the mixture into about 36 (1-inch) meatballs and arrange them on a baking sheet.

4. Bake the meatballs for about 15 minutes.

5. While the meatballs are baking, in a large skillet over medium-high heat, melt the coconut oil. Add the bell pepper and cook, stirring frequently, until it softens, about 4 minutes.

6. Add the pineapple, along with the juice, and cook until the pineapple is hot and the liquid is slightly reduced, about 5 minutes more.

7. In a small bowl, stir the arrowroot with a bit of water to make a slurry. Add the arrowroot mixture to the sauce, remove the skillet from the heat, and stir until the sauce thickens.

continued ▶

8. When meatballs are finished baking, add them to the skillet and toss to coat.

9. Transfer the meatballs and sauce to a serving dish, garnish them with the scallions, and serve them with toothpicks.

NUTRITIONAL INFORMATION PER SERVING: CALORIES 183 TOTAL FAT 9.0G SATURATED FAT 2.4G
TRANS FAT 0.0G SODIUM 90MG TOTAL CARBOHYDRATES 9.7G SUGARS 6.2G PROTEIN 19.2G

NOTES

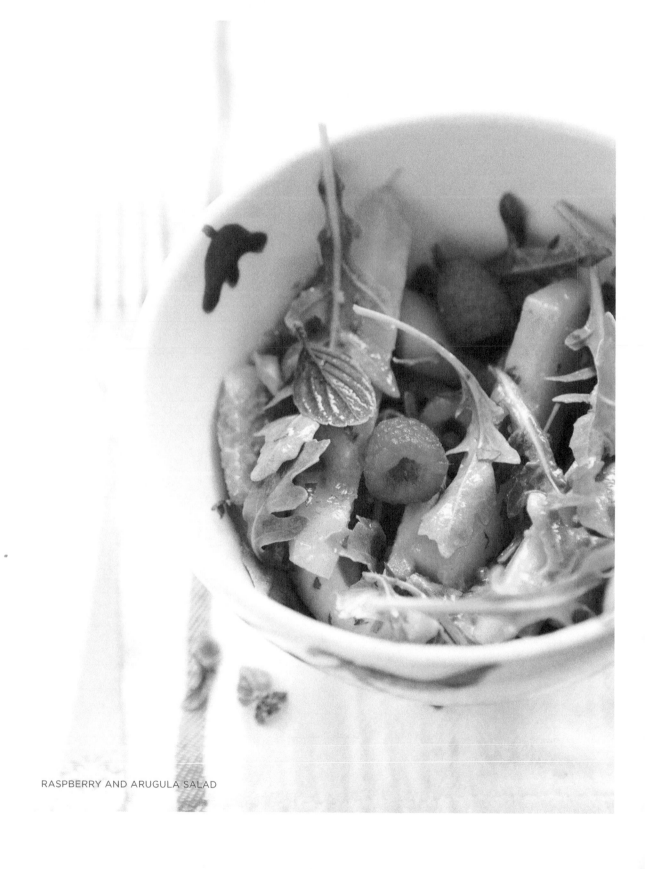

RASPBERRY AND ARUGULA SALAD

7

Salads

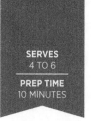

Asian-Style Slaw

This Asian-style slaw is different than American-style coleslaw not only in flavor but also in texture. It is made with a vinegar-based sauce rather than a creamy sauce, and the sesame oil and toasted sesame seeds make it distinctly Asian. To toast the sesame seeds, just put them in a dry heated pan and stir constantly until they start to brown.

Time-saving tip You can often find bagged, precut slaw mixes in the supermarket produce section. Look for one with Napa cabbage and carrots, but if you can't find that combination, any slaw mixture will do.

½ HEAD NAPA CABBAGE, THINLY SLICED

2 CARROTS, PEELED AND GRATED

¼ CUP DICED RED ONION

2 TABLESPOONS UNSEASONED RICE WINE VINEGAR

1 TABLESPOON APPLE CIDER VINEGAR

1 TABLESPOON FRESHLY SQUEEZED LIME JUICE

1 TABLESPOON HONEY

2 TEASPOONS GLUTEN-FREE SOY SAUCE

1 TEASPOON SESAME OIL

¼ CUP TOASTED SESAME SEEDS

1. In a large bowl, combine the cabbage, carrots, and onion, and toss to mix well.

2. In a small bowl, whisk together the rice wine vinegar, cider vinegar, lime juice, honey, soy sauce, sesame oil, and sesame seeds.

3. Pour the dressing over the cabbage mixture and toss to coat.

4. Cover the slaw with plastic wrap and place it in the refrigerator until ready to serve. It will store for up to 1 day.

5. Serve chilled.

NUTRITIONAL INFORMATION PER SERVING: CALORIES 116 TOTAL FAT 5.8G SATURATED FAT 0.8G TRANS FAT 0.0G SODIUM 588MG TOTAL CARBOHYDRATES 13.8G SUGARS 7.6G PROTEIN 4.5G

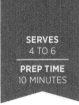

Creamy Coleslaw

If you are a fan of creamy coleslaw, this is definitely the recipe for you. This slaw makes a great accompaniment to any of the wing recipes (Spicy Buffalo Wings, page 98; Honey-Barbecue Wings, page 99; and Maple and Soy Wings, page 100) or Gluten-Free Fried Chicken (page 154).

½ HEAD NAPA CABBAGE,
   THINLY SLICED

½ HEAD RED CABBAGE,
   THINLY SLICED

4 CARROTS, PEELED AND GRATED

1 CUP MAYONNAISE, MADE WITH
   OLIVE OIL

½ CUP APPLE CIDER VINEGAR

¼ CUP HONEY

SALT

1. In a large bowl, combine the Napa cabbage, red cabbage, and carrots, and toss to mix well.

2. In a small bowl, whisk together the mayonnaise, vinegar, and honey. Season with salt and stir to combine well.

3. Pour the dressing over the slaw and toss well to coat.

4. Cover the slaw with plastic wrap, and refrigerate it until ready to serve. It will store for up to 1 day.

5. Serve chilled.

NUTRITIONAL INFORMATION PER SERVING: CALORIES 361 TOTAL FAT 19.9G SATURATED FAT 2.9G
TRANS FAT 0.0G SODIUM 585MG TOTAL CARBOHYDRATES 45.2G SUGARS 28.4G PROTEIN 3.8G

Mango-Cucumber Salad

This salad is incredibly simple to make, and it is the perfect dish to enjoy on a hot day. Serve it as a light and refreshing side dish alongside grilled meats, wings, or fried chicken. If the mango isn't quite ripe enough, add an extra touch of honey.

2 SEEDLESS CUCUMBERS, PEELED AND
    THINLY SLICED

1 MANGO, PEELED, PITTED, AND DICED

2 TABLESPOONS MINCED RED ONION

1 TABLESPOON UNSEASONED RICE
    WINE VINEGAR

1 TABLESPOON HONEY

1. In a serving bowl, combine the cucumbers, mango, and onion.

2. Toss the salad with the vinegar and honey until coated.

3. Serve the salad at room temperature or chilled.

NUTRITIONAL INFORMATION PER SERVING: CALORIES 55   TOTAL FAT 0.3G   SATURATED FAT 0.0G
TRANS FAT 0.0G   SODIUM 3MG   TOTAL CARBOHYDRATES 13.5G   SUGARS 8.2G   PROTEIN 0.9G

Summer Squash Salad

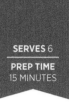

If you grow your own vegetables in the summer, you've probably been drowning in zucchini. This recipe is a great way to use up some of that bountiful produce. If you don't grow your own, visit your local farmers' market anytime from June through August and you'll likely have plenty of varieties of summer squash to choose from.

Ingredient tip Choose any type of soft-skinned summer squash, such as regular zucchini, yellow zucchini, crookneck, or pattypan squash, for this salad.

1 ZUCCHINI, THINLY SLICED

2 SUMMER SQUASH OF YOUR CHOICE,
THINLY SLICED

2 TABLESPOONS CHOPPED
FRESH BASIL

2 TABLESPOONS EXTRA-VIRGIN
OLIVE OIL

1 TABLESPOON FRESHLY SQUEEZED
LEMON JUICE

1 TEASPOON BALSAMIC VINEGAR

PINCH SALT

PINCH FRESHLY GROUND BLACK PEPPER

2 TABLESPOONS SLICED ALMONDS

1. In a serving bowl, combine the zucchini, summer squash, and basil.

2. In a small bowl, whisk together the olive oil, lemon juice, and vinegar. Season the dressing with salt and pepper.

3. Toss the vegetables with the dressing to coat.

4. Sprinkle the salad with the sliced almonds. Serve the salad at room temperature or briefly chilled.

NUTRITIONAL INFORMATION PER SERVING: CALORIES 68   TOTAL FAT 5.9G   SATURATED FAT 0.8G
TRANS FAT 0.0G   SODIUM 38MG   TOTAL CARBOHYDRATES 3.8G   SUGARS 1.8G   PROTEIN 1.7G

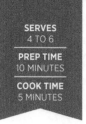

SERVES
4 TO 6

PREP TIME
10 MINUTES

COOK TIME
5 MINUTES

Asparagus and Avocado Salad

Made with tender asparagus and creamy avocado, this salad is surprisingly hearty. With the pale green hues of asparagus, avocado, and basil punctuated by bright red cherry tomatoes, this salad is as pretty as it is delicious.

Ingredient tip Contrary to popular belief, thin asparagus spears aren't necessarily more desirable than fat ones. It's just a matter of personal preference and aesthetics. Whichever type you choose, snap off the woody, fibrous ends by bending the asparagus stalk near the bottom. The spear will snap and break where the woody part begins.

1 POUND ASPARAGUS SPEARS

1 CUP HALVED CHERRY TOMATOES

1 AVOCADO, PEELED, PITTED, AND
    CHOPPED

¼ CUP PACKED FRESH BASIL LEAVES

¼ CUP EXTRA-VIRGIN OLIVE OIL

2 TEASPOONS FRESHLY SQUEEZED
    LEMON JUICE

1 TEASPOON BALSAMIC VINEGAR

1 TEASPOON DIJON MUSTARD

SALT

FRESHLY GROUND BLACK PEPPER

1. Trim the bottoms from the asparagus and cut the spears into 2-inch segments.

2. Place the asparagus in a steamer basket inside a large lidded saucepan and add about 2 inches of water.

3. Over medium-high heat, bring the water to boil, cover, and steam the asparagus for about 5 minutes, until just fork tender.

4. Drain the asparagus and place it in a serving bowl. Add the tomatoes, avocado, and basil.

5. In a small bowl, whisk together the olive oil, lemon juice, vinegar, and mustard. Pour the dressing over the salad and toss to coat.

6. Season the salad with salt and pepper. Serve warm.

NUTRITIONAL INFORMATION PER SERVING: CALORIES 246 TOTAL FAT 22.6G SATURATED FAT 3.9G
TRANS FAT 0.0G SODIUM 65MG TOTAL CARBOHYDRATES 11.4G SUGARS 3.9G PROTEIN 4.1G

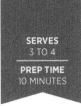
Fennel, Basil, and Orange Salad

Fennel has a distinctive but delicate flavor that is similar to licorice. The fennel and orange combination is classic, and it shines in this simple and refreshing salad. For variety or to make more of a substantial salad that can serve as a meal, add chopped kalamata olives or feta cheese to the mix.

Cooking tip Raw fennel is fairly fibrous and is most enjoyable to eat when it is sliced very thin. Use a mandoline to get paper-thin slices. If you don't have a mandoline, use a very sharp knife and a steady hand. Resist the urge to slice the fennel bulb in the food processor, as that will produce slices that are too thick.

1 BULB FENNEL, THINLY SLICED

¼ CUP CHOPPED FRESH BASIL

2 NAVEL ORANGES, PEELED AND SECTIONED

2 TABLESPOONS EXTRA-VIRGIN OLIVE OIL

2 TABLESPOONS RED WINE VINEGAR

1 TEASPOON HONEY

SALT

FRESHLY GROUND BLACK PEPPER

2 TABLESPOONS RAISINS OR DRIED CRANBERRIES

1. In a serving bowl, combine the fennel, basil, and oranges.

2. In a small bowl, whisk together the olive oil, vinegar, and honey. Season the dressing with salt and pepper, then pour it over the salad and toss to coat.

3. Sprinkle the raisins onto the salad.

4. Chill the salad until ready to serve. It will store for up to 1 day.

NUTRITIONAL INFORMATION PER SERVING: CALORIES 142 TOTAL FAT 7.3G SATURATED FAT 1.0G
TRANS FAT 0.0G **SODIUM** 70MG **TOTAL CARBOHYDRATES** 20.2G **SUGARS** 12.7G **PROTEIN** 1.8G

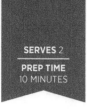
Raspberry and Arugula Salad

This simple green salad is studded with bright red raspberries and dressed with a sweet and tangy raspberry vinaigrette. Peppery and slightly bitter fresh arugula is the perfect backdrop for the sweet, juicy fruit. Don't be tempted to leave out the dry mustard, as it adds just the right hint of spice to balance the sweetness of the dressing.

Ingredient tip If you don't have fresh raspberries, substitute fresh strawberries and strawberry jam.

4 CUPS FRESH ARUGULA

½ CANTALOUPE, SLICED INTO WEDGES

1 SCALLION, THINLY SLICED

2 TABLESPOONS EXTRA-VIRGIN
   OLIVE OIL

1 TABLESPOON APPLE CIDER VINEGAR

1 TABLESPOON RASPBERRY JAM

PINCH DRY MUSTARD POWDER

2 CUPS FRESH RASPBERRIES

1. In a salad bowl, combine the arugula, cantaloupe, and scallion and toss well.

2. In a small bowl, whisk together the olive oil, vinegar, jam, and mustard powder until well combined.

3. Pour the dressing over the salad and toss to coat.

4. Top the salad with the fresh raspberries to serve.

NUTRITIONAL INFORMATION PER SERVING: **CALORIES** 224 **TOTAL FAT** 15.1G **SATURATED FAT** 2.0G
TRANS FAT 0.0G **SODIUM** 14MG **TOTAL CARBOHYDRATES** 23.3G **SUGARS** 11.0G **PROTEIN** 2.8G

Mixed Spring Greens Salad

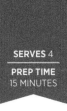

Full of the flavors of spring, this salad is loaded with fresh vegetables, including salad greens, fresh basil, sugar snap peas, and zucchini. For a bit of crunch, top it with a sprinkling of toasted pine nuts or chopped toasted hazelnuts.

6 CUPS MIXED SPRING GREENS

2 SCALLIONS, THINLY SLICED

1 CUP SUGAR SNAP PEAS, STRINGS
    REMOVED

1 ZUCCHINI, THINLY SLICED

¼ CUP CHOPPED FRESH BASIL

2 TABLESPOONS EXTRA-VIRGIN
    OLIVE OIL

1 TABLESPOON UNSEASONED RICE
    WINE VINEGAR

1 TEASPOON FRESHLY SQUEEZED
    LEMON JUICE

1 TEASPOON HONEY

PINCH GROUND GINGER

1. In a salad bowl, combine the spring greens, scallions, snap peas, zucchini, and basil, and stir to combine.

2. In a small bowl, whisk together the olive oil, vinegar, lemon juice, honey, and ginger.

3. Pour the dressing over the salad and toss to coat. Or chill the salad up to 4 hours and pour the dressing over the salad just before serving.

NUTRITIONAL INFORMATION PER SERVING: CALORIES 96 TOTAL FAT 7.1G SATURATED FAT 1.0G
TRANS FAT 0.0G SODIUM 17MG TOTAL CARBOHYDRATES 7.6G SUGARS 3.1G PROTEIN 2.1G

Spinach Salad with Lemon-Balsamic Dressing

This simple spinach salad is dressed up with a bright, citrusy vinaigrette. One taste and you'll wonder why you ever bought commercial salad dressings (which often contain hidden gluten) when such delicious dressing is so easy to make at home.

6 CUPS GENTLY PACKED FRESH
   BABY SPINACH
1 CARROT, SHREDDED
½ RED ONION, THINLY SLICED
3 TABLESPOONS EXTRA-VIRGIN OLIVE OIL
2 TABLESPOONS FRESHLY SQUEEZED
   LEMON JUICE

2 TABLESPOONS BALSAMIC VINEGAR
1 TEASPOON HONEY
1 TEASPOON DIJON MUSTARD
CHOPPED NUTS OR RAISINS, FOR
   GARNISH (OPTIONAL)

1. In a salad bowl, toss together the spinach, carrot, and onion.

2. In a small bowl, whisk together the olive oil, lemon juice, vinegar, honey, and mustard until well combined.

3. Toss the dressing with the salad just before serving.

4. Garnish with chopped nuts or raisins (if using).

NUTRITIONAL INFORMATION PER SERVING: **CALORIES** 122 **TOTAL FAT** 10.8G **SATURATED FAT** 1.6G **TRANS FAT** 0.0G **SODIUM** 62MG **TOTAL CARBOHYDRATES** 6.2G **DIETARY FIBER** 1.7G **SUGARS** 3.2G **PROTEIN** 1.6G

Apple and Radicchio Salad

SERVES 4

PREP TIME
10 MINUTES

Radicchio is a leafy vegetable—a bright pinkish-purplish-reddish chicory with a bitter bite—that you've probably seen as a supporting actor in mixed salads. In this recipe, it becomes the star. Its bitter edge is balanced by the sweetness of the apples. Toasted walnuts add the perfect nutty crunch.

1 HEAD RADICCHIO, THINLY SLICED

3 CUPS GENTLY PACKED
   SPRING GREENS

1 APPLE, PEELED, CORED, AND CUT
   INTO MATCHSTICKS

2 TABLESPOONS EXTRA-VIRGIN
   OLIVE OIL

1½ TABLESPOONS BALSAMIC VINEGAR

1 TEASPOON RED WINE VINEGAR

SALT

FRESHLY GROUND BLACK PEPPER

3 TABLESPOONS CHOPPED TOASTED
   WALNUTS, FOR GARNISH

1. In a salad bowl, combine the radicchio, greens, and apple.

2. In a small bowl, whisk together the olive oil, balsamic vinegar, and red wine vinegar. Season the dressing with salt and pepper. Whisk to combine well.

3. Toss the dressing with the salad to coat.

4. Serve the salad garnished with chopped walnuts.

NUTRITIONAL INFORMATION PER SERVING: **CALORIES** 133   **TOTAL FAT** 10.5G   **SATURATED FAT** 1.2G
TRANS FAT 0.0G   **SODIUM** 70MG   **TOTAL CARBOHYDRATES** 9.2G   **SUGARS** 5.0G   **PROTEIN** 2.1G

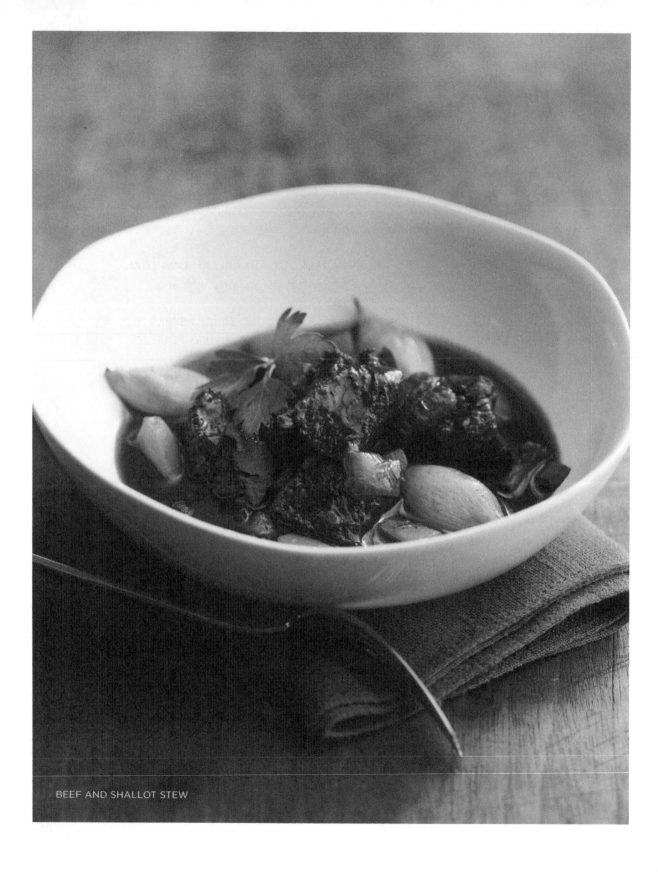

BEEF AND SHALLOT STEW

8

Soups, Stews, and Chilies

SERVES
4 TO 6

PREP TIME
10 MINUTES

COOK TIME
20 MINUTES

Cream of Cauliflower Soup

This creamy white soup may look a bit plain in the bowl, but it has a rich, complex flavor. Frozen, thawed cauliflower will cook a bit faster than fresh, plus you can keep a bag in your freezer so that you can whip up this soup any time you please. The other ingredients are all pantry staples.

3½ CUPS UNSWEETENED
    COCONUT MILK
1 TEASPOON MINCED GARLIC
1 CUP CHOPPED YELLOW ONION

1 (16-OUNCE) BAG FROZEN
    CAULIFLOWER FLORETS, THAWED
2 TEASPOONS CURRY POWDER
SALT
FRESHLY GROUND BLACK PEPPER

1. In a large saucepan over medium heat, warm ½ cup of the coconut milk.

2. Stir in the garlic and onion and cook for about 5 minutes, until softened.

3. Add the cauliflower, the remaining 3 cups of coconut milk, and curry powder. Season the soup with salt and pepper. Stir to combine.

4. Increase the heat to medium-high, bring the soup to a boil, then reduce the heat to low and simmer, covered, for about 15 minutes, or until the cauliflower is very tender.

5. Remove the soup from the heat and purée it in a blender or use an immersion blender to purée it in the pot. Serve hot.

NUTRITIONAL INFORMATION PER SERVING: CALORIES 84   TOTAL FAT 4.2G   SATURATED FAT 3.5G
TRANS FAT 0.0G   SODIUM 87MG   TOTAL CARBOHYDRATES 11.3G   SUGARS 4.9G   PROTEIN 2.6G

Cream of Mushroom Soup

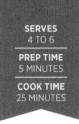

SERVES
4 TO 6

PREP TIME
5 MINUTES

COOK TIME
25 MINUTES

Cream of mushroom soup is a classic that's quick and simple to make but tastes a bit decadent. This version is enriched with heavy cream and flavored with fresh thyme. While many commercial versions are thickened with wheat flour, this recipe uses cornstarch to stay gluten-free.

1 POUND ASSORTED MUSHROOMS, VERY FINELY MINCED

1 TABLESPOON FRESHLY SQUEEZED LEMON JUICE

1 TABLESPOON EXTRA-VIRGIN OLIVE OIL

¼ CUP SLICED SHALLOTS

1 TEASPOON DRIED THYME

SALT

FRESHLY GROUND BLACK PEPPER

2 CUPS GLUTEN-FREE CHICKEN BROTH

1 CUP HEAVY CREAM

1 TABLESPOON WATER

1 TEASPOON CORNSTARCH

1. In a medium bowl, stir together the mushrooms and lemon juice.

2. Heat the olive oil in a large saucepan over medium-high heat. Stir in the shallots and cook, stirring often, for 2 minutes, or until they are slightly softened.

3. Add the mushroom mixture and thyme, season with salt and pepper, and stir to combine.

4. Cook, stirring often, for 6 minutes, or until the mushrooms release their liquid and it cooks off.

5. Stir in the chicken broth and heavy cream. Increase the heat to medium-high and bring the soup to a boil.

6. Reduce the heat to low and simmer, covered, for 15 minutes.

7. In a small bowl, add the water and cornstarch and stir until combined.

8. Whisk the cornstarch into the mushroom soup, then turn up the heat to medium-high and simmer for another 2 minutes, until thickened. Serve hot.

NUTRITIONAL INFORMATION PER SERVING: CALORIES 177 TOTAL FAT 15.2G SATURATED FAT 7.5G
TRANS FAT 0.0G SODIUM 116MG TOTAL CARBOHYDRATES 8.1G SUGARS 2.5G PROTEIN 5.0G

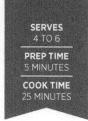

SERVES
4 TO 6

PREP TIME
5 MINUTES

COOK TIME
25 MINUTES

Butternut Squash Soup

Butternut squash soup is naturally gluten-free. This version is delightfully simple, but you can dress it up any way you like. Add a dash of cumin and ground chipotle for a spicy Mexican-style soup. Try a spoonful of curry powder, a bit of cayenne pepper, and a dollop of yogurt for an Indian flavor. Or go for a North African style with cinnamon, clove, and *ras el hanout* (a Moroccan spice blend).

Time-saving tip Peeling an uncooked butternut squash can be difficult, although a sharp carrot peeler will do the job. Make it easier by microwaving the squash for 5 to 10 minutes before peeling.

1½ TABLESPOONS EXTRA-VIRGIN
    OLIVE OIL

1 CUP DICED WHITE ONION

½ CUP DICED CELERY

½ CUP DICED CARROT

4 CUPS PEELED, DICED
    BUTTERNUT SQUASH

4 CUPS GLUTEN-FREE CHICKEN BROTH

¼ TEASPOON DRIED THYME

SALT

FRESHLY GROUND BLACK PEPPER

1. Heat the olive oil in a large soup pot over medium-high heat.

2. Add the onion, celery, and carrot, and cook, stirring often, for 4 minutes, or until the onions begin to turn translucent.

3. Stir in the butternut squash, chicken broth, and thyme. Season with salt and pepper.

4. Bring the soup to a boil. Reduce the heat to medium and simmer for about 20 minutes, until the squash is tender.

5. Remove the soup from the heat and purée it in a blender or use an immersion blender to purée it in the pot. Serve hot.

NUTRITIONAL INFORMATION PER SERVING: **CALORIES** 133 **TOTAL FAT** 5.9G **SATURATED FAT** 0.8G
TRANS FAT 0.0G **SODIUM** 175MG **TOTAL CARBOHYDRATES** 20.6G **SUGARS** 14.3G **PROTEIN** 1.7G

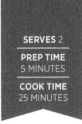

Chicken "Noodle" Soup

This recipe doesn't actually contain any noodles; julienned zucchini takes the place of pasta in this classic recipe. If you don't have a julienne slicer, jut cut the zucchini into matchsticks. You could substitute any summer squash for the zucchini. If you'd like a heartier soup, add a handful of cooked gluten-free pasta just before serving.

4 CUPS GLUTEN-FREE CHICKEN BROTH
1 TEASPOON DRIED OREGANO
SALT
FRESHLY GROUND BLACK PEPPER
1 CARROT, DICED

1 CELERY STALK, DICED
½ CUP DICED WHITE ONION
1 ZUCCHINI, PEELED WITH A
     JULIENNE SLICER

1. In a large stockpot, pour in the chicken broth. Add the oregano and season the broth with salt and pepper. Stir to combine and bring the broth to a boil over medium-high heat.

2. Reduce the heat to medium, and add the carrot, celery, and onion. Simmer the mixture for 10 to 15 minutes, until the carrot is tender.

3. Stir in the julienned zucchini and simmer for 3 to 5 minutes more, until the zucchini is tender. Serve hot.

NUTRITIONAL INFORMATION PER SERVING: CALORIES 74   TOTAL FAT 1.3G   SATURATED FAT 0.0G
TRANS FAT 0.0G   SODIUM 345MG   TOTAL CARBOHYDRATES 13.7G   SUGARS 6.6G   PROTEIN 3.8G

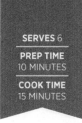
Thai Chicken Coconut Soup

This Thai soup is easy to prepare and is full of exotic flavor. If you like your soup a little spicier, add a minced Thai or jalapeño pepper along with the garlic and onion or a pinch of cayenne or red pepper flakes along with the chicken.

1 TABLESPOON EXTRA-VIRGIN
   OLIVE OIL
1 TEASPOON MINCED GARLIC
½ CUP CHOPPED WHITE ONION
4 CUPS GLUTEN-FREE CHICKEN BROTH
2 (14-OUNCE) CANS COCONUT MILK
2 CUPS DICED SHIITAKE MUSHROOMS
1 HEAD BROCCOLI, CHOPPED

1 POUND BONELESS SKINLESS
   CHICKEN BREAST, CHOPPED
2½ TABLESPOONS FRESHLY SQUEEZED
   LIME JUICE
2 TABLESPOONS GLUTEN-FREE THAI
   FISH SAUCE
2 TEASPOONS CURRY PASTE

1. Heat the olive oil in a large soup pot over medium heat.

2. Stir in the garlic and onion and cook for 5 minutes, stirring, until the onion softens.

3. Add the chicken broth and coconut milk, increase the heat to medium-high, and bring the mixture almost to a boil.

4. Reduce the heat to medium and simmer, then stir in the mushrooms and broccoli. Cook the mixture for 2 minutes, stirring often.

5. Stir in the chicken and cook for 3 minutes.

6. In a small bowl, whisk together the lime juice, fish sauce, and curry paste, then stir it into the soup.

7. Cook the soup, stirring occasionally, for 2 minutes, until the soup is heated through. Serve hot.

NUTRITIONAL INFORMATION PER SERVING: CALORIES 509   TOTAL FAT 40.9G   SATURATED FAT 29.8G
TRANS FAT 0.0G   SODIUM 744MG   TOTAL CARBOHYDRATES 12.3G   SUGARS 6.1G   PROTEIN 27.6G

Moroccan Vegetable Stew

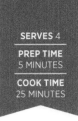

By using ready-to-cook vegetables and canned beans, this hearty stew can be ready in the time it would take to stop for takeout. Cinnamon, cumin, and cloves give this stew a distinctly North African flavor, and raisins add a pleasant sweetness. Serve this stew with a dollop of plain yogurt, if you like.

2 TABLESPOONS EXTRA-VIRGIN
   OLIVE OIL
2 SHALLOTS, DICED
1 (15-OUNCE) CAN CHICKPEAS,
   DRAINED, WITH LIQUID RESERVED
1 LARGE POTATO, PEELED AND CUT
   INTO ¾-INCH CUBES
1¾ CUPS BABY CARROTS
⅓ CUP RAISINS

1½ TEASPOONS GROUND CUMIN
½ TEASPOON CINNAMON
½ TEASPOON SALT
½ TEASPOON FRESHLY GROUND
   BLACK PEPPER
PINCH GROUND CLOVES
2 CUPS BABY SPINACH LEAVES
FRESHLY SQUEEZED JUICE OF
   ½ LEMON

1. Heat the olive oil in large skillet over medium-high heat. Add the shallots and cook, stirring, until they soften, about 5 minutes.

2. Add the reserved chickpea liquid, potato, carrots, raisins, cumin, cinnamon, salt, pepper, and cloves. Cook the mixture, stirring occasionally, and bring it to a simmer. Reduce the heat to medium-low and simmer, covered, for 8 minutes.

3. Add half the chickpeas, cover, and cook about 5 minutes more. The potato and carrots should be tender but not soft.

4. In a bowl, mash the remaining chickpeas with a fork and then stir them into the stew. Simmer for 2 minutes, or until the stew is heated through.

5. Stir in the spinach and cook for about 2 minutes more, until the spinach is wilted.

6. Stir in the lemon juice and serve hot.

NUTRITIONAL INFORMATION PER SERVING: CALORIES 564 TOTAL FAT 13.8G SATURATED FAT 1.7G
TRANS FAT 0.0G SODIUM 353MG TOTAL CARBOHYDRATES 91.7G SUGARS 18.6G PROTEIN 23.5G

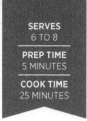

SERVES
6 TO 8

PREP TIME
5 MINUTES

COOK TIME
25 MINUTES

Vegetarian Eggplant Stew

This tomato-based stew, loaded with tender vegetables and flavored with turmeric and garlic, is similar in flavor to a ratatouille. This version may not be strictly traditional, but it is quick to make and very satisfying. Serve it hot on a chilly evening or enjoy it as a hearty lunch.

Cooking tip If you have the time, sprinkle salt on the cut eggplant and let it drain on paper towels or in a colander for 20 to 30 minutes. This will draw out any bitterness. Rinse off the salt and pat the eggplant dry before cooking.

4 TABLESPOONS EXTRA-VIRGIN
    OLIVE OIL

1½ POUNDS EGGPLANT, PEELED AND
    FINELY DICED

1 YELLOW ONION, FINELY CHOPPED

1 RED BELL PEPPER, FINELY CHOPPED

2 ZUCCHINI, DICED

½ TEASPOON GROUND TURMERIC

1 TEASPOON MINCED GARLIC

1 CUP TOMATO SAUCE

1 CUP WATER

1 (15-OUNCE) CAN CHICKPEAS,
    DRAINED AND RINSED

1. Heat 2 tablespoons of olive oil in a large skillet over medium-high heat.

2. When the oil is hot, add the eggplant and stir well. Reduce the heat immediately to medium and cook for about 6 minutes, stirring often, until the eggplant is tender.

3. Meanwhile, heat the remaining 2 tablespoons of olive oil in a Dutch oven over medium-high heat. Stir in the onion, bell pepper, and zucchini, and cook for 4 minutes, stirring often, until the onion is tender.

4. Stir in the turmeric and garlic and cook for 30 seconds.

5. Add the tomato sauce, water, chickpeas, and cooked eggplant, and bring the mixture to a boil.

6. Reduce the heat to medium-low and simmer for 15 minutes, or until the vegetables are tender. Serve hot.

NUTRITIONAL INFORMATION PER SERVING: CALORIES 401 TOTAL FAT 14.2G SATURATED FAT 1.8G
TRANS FAT 0.0G SODIUM 242MG TOTAL CARBOHYDRATES 57.0G SUGARS 14.7G PROTEIN 16.5G

Curried Chicken Stew

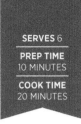

SERVES 6

PREP TIME
10 MINUTES

COOK TIME
20 MINUTES

Making this flavorful chicken curry is much quicker than ordering and picking up takeout. Better still, it's not loaded with fat or empty calories. Serve it with Grain-Free Flatbread (page 44) or brown rice to soak up the tasty sauce.

Time-saving tip Instead of buying whole chicken breasts and cutting them up, get boneless chicken breast tenders. They come in small strips that can be added to the pan whole.

2 TABLESPOONS EXTRA-VIRGIN OLIVE OIL

1½ POUNDS BONELESS SKINLESS CHICKEN BREAST, CHOPPED

1 YELLOW ONION, SLICED

1½ CUPS WATER

1 CUP SLICED CARROTS

2 CUPS QUARTERED NEW POTATOES

1 CUP FROZEN PEAS

1 CUP HALF-AND-HALF

1 CUP GLUTEN-FREE CHICKEN BROTH

1 GLUTEN-FREE CHICKEN BOUILLON CUBE

1 TABLESPOON CURRY POWDER

1. Heat the olive oil in a large, heavy saucepan over medium heat.

2. Stir in the chicken and onion and cook, stirring often, for 2 to 3 minutes, until the onion softens.

3. Add the water, carrots, and potatoes, and cook for 4 to 6 minutes, until the mixture comes to a boil.

4. Stir in the peas, half-and-half, chicken broth, bouillon cube, and curry powder, crushing the bouillon cube until it dissolves.

5. Reduce the heat to medium-low and simmer for 10 to 15 minutes, until the vegetables are tender. Serve hot.

NUTRITIONAL INFORMATION PER SERVING: CALORIES 369 TOTAL FAT 18.0G SATURATED FAT 5.9G
TRANS FAT 0.0G SODIUM 169MG TOTAL CARBOHYDRATES 14.3G SUGARS 3.4G PROTEIN 36.5G

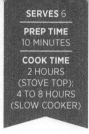

SERVES 6

PREP TIME
10 MINUTES

COOK TIME
2 HOURS
(STOVE TOP);
4 TO 8 HOURS
(SLOW COOKER)

Beef and Shallot Stew

Classic beef stew—drenched in a rich, meaty gravy and studded with carrots and shallots—is a family favorite, but most recipes involve tossing the meat with flour to thicken the gravy. This recipe uses almond flour; if you avoid nuts, you could use gluten-free all-purpose flour (homemade recipe on page 32) instead. This recipe can be cooked either in a slow cooker or on the stove top.

Time-saving tip To shave several minutes off your prep time, ask your butcher to do it for you. They have super-sharp knives and lots of practice.

2 POUNDS BEEF STEW MEAT, CUBED

SALT

FRESHLY GROUND BLACK PEPPER

2 TABLESPOONS ALMOND FLOUR

2 TABLESPOONS EXTRA-VIRGIN OLIVE OIL

8–10 GARLIC CLOVES

10 SHALLOTS, PEELED,
BULBS SEPARATED

1 CUP SLICED CARROTS

2 CUPS GLUTEN-FREE BEEF BROTH

1 TEASPOON DRIED THYME

1 TEASPOON DRIED SAGE

1. Season the beef with salt and pepper, then place it in a plastic bag. Add the almond flour, seal the bag shut, and shake it well to coat.

2. Heat the olive oil in a medium skillet over medium-high heat and add the beef and garlic cloves. Cook for 3 to 4 minutes, turning occasionally, until it is lightly browned on all sides.

3. If using a slow cooker, transfer the meat to the slow cooker (use one with a 6-quart capacity). Stir in the shallots, carrots, beef broth, thyme, and sage. Cover and cook on low heat for 6 to 8 hours or on high heat for 4 to 5 hours, until the meat and vegetables are tender.

4. If cooking on the stove top, heat a 6-quart Dutch oven or large stockpot over medium heat. Add the meat, shallots, carrots, beef broth, thyme, and sage, and bring the mixture to a boil. Cover, reduce the heat to low, and simmer, stirring occasionally, until the meat is very tender, about 2 hours. Serve hot.

NUTRITIONAL INFORMATION PER SERVING: CALORIES 403 TOTAL FAT 18.8G SATURATED FAT 4.6G
TRANS FAT 0.0G SODIUM 333MG TOTAL CARBOHYDRATES 7.7G SUGARS 3.1G PROTEIN 49.0G

SERVES 6 TO 8

PREP TIME
10 MINUTES

COOK TIME
3 HOURS
(STOVE TOP);
8 TO 10 HOURS
(SLOW COOKER)

Three-Bean Chili

Beans are an excellent source of fiber and are also full of protein. Here, black beans, pinto beans, kidney beans, and lentils pack this vegetarian chili full of powerful nutrients. Serve with grated cheese, sour cream, diced onion, and other toppings that guests can add to their own bowls. This recipe can be cooked either in a slow cooker or on the stove top.

1 (15-OUNCE) CAN BLACK BEANS,
    DRAINED AND RINSED
1 (15-OUNCE) CAN RED KIDNEY BEANS,
    DRAINED AND RINSED
1 (15-OUNCE) CAN PINTO BEANS,
    DRAINED AND RINSED
1 CUP DRIED LENTILS
3 CUPS GLUTEN-FREE CHICKEN BROTH

2 TABLESPOONS CHILI POWDER
½ TEASPOON GROUND CUMIN
¼ TEASPOON GROUND CORIANDER
1 (10-OUNCE) CAN DICED TOMATOES,
    WITH JUICE
1 (15-OUNCE) CAN TOMATO SAUCE
SALT
FRESHLY GROUND BLACK PEPPER

1. If using a slow cooker, combine the black beans, kidney beans, pinto beans, lentils, chicken broth, chili powder, cumin, and coriander in the slow cooker, and stir to combine. Cover and cook on low heat for 8 to 10 hours, until the lentils are soft.

2. If cooking on the stove top, heat a large Dutch oven or stockpot over medium heat. Add the black beans, kidney beans, pinto beans, lentils, chicken broth, chili powder, cumin, and coriander, and bring to a simmer. Cover, reduce the heat to low, and simmer, stirring occasionally, until the lentils are soft, about 3 hours.

3. Stir in the diced tomatoes and tomato sauce and season with salt and pepper.

4. Cook for 5 minutes on high heat, until it has thickened slightly. Serve hot.

NUTRITIONAL INFORMATION PER SERVING: CALORIES 661   TOTAL FAT 2.9G   SATURATED FAT 0.5G
TRANS FAT 0.0G   **SODIUM** 379MG   **TOTAL CARBOHYDRATES** 119.5G   **SUGARS** 7.6G   **PROTEIN** 42.7G

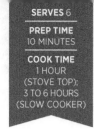

SERVES 6

PREP TIME
10 MINUTES

COOK TIME
1 HOUR
(STOVE TOP);
3 TO 6 HOURS
(SLOW COOKER)

Spicy Turkey Chili

If you are looking for a hot and hearty recipe to warm you up on a cold night, look no further than this spicy turkey chili with black beans. To serve, ladle it into soup bowls and offer grated cheese, sour cream, (gluten-free) tortilla chips, guacamole, diced onion, cilantro, or whatever other toppings appeal to you. This recipe can be cooked either in a slow cooker or on the stove top.

Ingredient tip If you don't have black beans, substitute a different type. Pinto beans, kidney beans, or even cannellini beans would all work well.

1½ POUNDS BONELESS SKINLESS
    TURKEY BREAST, CHOPPED
1 TABLESPOON MINCED GARLIC
2 SERRANO CHILES, SEEDED
    AND MINCED
1 YELLOW ONION, CHOPPED
1 (28-OUNCE) CAN DICED TOMATOES,
    WITH JUICE

2 TABLESPOONS CHILI POWDER
¼ TEASPOON GROUND CUMIN
2 (15-OUNCE) CANS BLACK BEANS,
    DRAINED AND RINSED
2 TEASPOONS APPLE CIDER VINEGAR
1 TEASPOON SALT
PINCH CAYENNE PEPPER

1. If using a slow cooker, combine the turkey, garlic, chiles, onion, tomatoes, chili powder, cumin, beans, vinegar, salt, and cayenne pepper in the slow cooker, and stir well. Cover and cook on high heat for 3 hours or on low heat for about 6 hours, until the turkey is cooked through.

2. If cooking on the stove top, heat a large Dutch oven or stockpot over medium heat. Add the turkey, garlic, chiles, onion, tomatoes, chili powder, cumin, beans, vinegar, salt, and cayenne pepper. Cover, reduce the heat to low, and simmer, stirring occasionally, until the turkey is cooked through, about 1 hour.

3. Serve hot.

NUTRITIONAL INFORMATION PER SERVING: CALORIES 636 TOTAL FAT 3.2G SATURATED FAT 0.6G
TRANS FAT 0.0G SODIUM 482MG TOTAL CARBOHYDRATES 97.2G SUGARS 7.4G PROTEIN 60.5G

NOTES

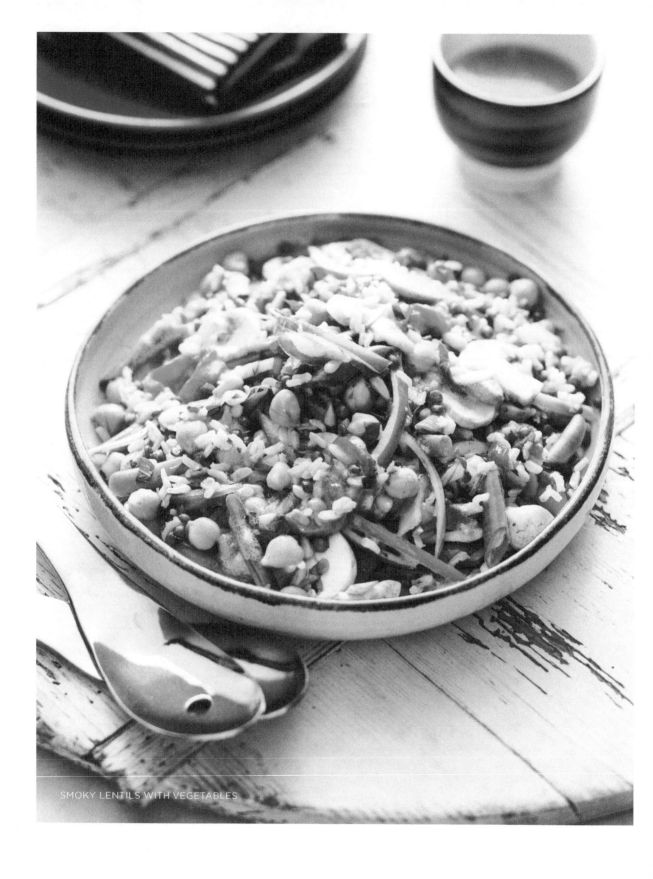

SMOKY LENTILS WITH VEGETABLES

9

Vegetarian Entrées

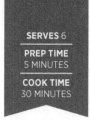
Baked Macaroni and Cheese

These days there are plenty of gluten-free pastas to choose from, including those made from brown rice, corn, and even quinoa. Use whatever version you prefer. This recipe uses almond milk and vegan cheese, but if you eat dairy, feel free to substitute the real thing.

Ingredient tip If you don't have gluten-free bread crumbs on hand, use crushed gluten-free crackers instead.

12 OUNCES GLUTEN-FREE
    MACARONI PASTA

NONSTICK COOKING SPRAY

2½ TABLESPOONS EXTRA-VIRGIN
    OLIVE OIL

2½ TABLESPOONS WHITE RICE FLOUR

2½ CUPS UNSWEETENED ALMOND MILK

2 CUPS SHREDDED VEGAN CHEESE

½ TEASPOON SALT

¼ TEASPOON GROUND NUTMEG

1 CUP GLUTEN-FREE BREAD CRUMBS

1. Bring a large pot of salted water to a boil. Add the macaroni and cook for 6 minutes, or until it softens but is still firm to the bite. Drain and set aside.

2. Preheat the oven to 375°F.

3. Coat a casserole dish with nonstick cooking spray.

4. Meanwhile, heat the olive oil in a medium saucepan over medium-high heat and whisk in the rice flour. Cook for 15 seconds, whisking constantly.

5. Gradually add the almond milk in a steady stream, whisking to create a paste.

6. Bring the mixture to a simmer, then reduce the heat to medium-low. Stir in the vegan cheese, salt, and nutmeg, and stir well.

7. Cook the cheese mixture for 3 to 5 minutes, stirring often, until it is melted and smooth.

8. Stir the cooked pasta into the cheese sauce and spoon it into the casserole dish.

9. Sprinkle the macaroni and cheese with the bread crumbs, and bake it for 20 minutes, or until the cheese is hot and bubbling. Serve hot.

NUTRITIONAL INFORMATION PER SERVING: CALORIES 611 TOTAL FAT 28.1G SATURATED FAT 12.5G TRANS FAT 0.0G SODIUM 1,104MG TOTAL CARBOHYDRATES 78.1G SUGARS 1.9G PROTEIN 9.5G

Dairy-Free Stuffed Pasta Shells

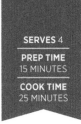

SERVES 4

PREP TIME
15 MINUTES

COOK TIME
25 MINUTES

If you avoid dairy in addition to gluten, you'll appreciate this dairy-free stuffed pasta recipe. Gluten-free pasta shells are filled with a mixture of pork sausage, spinach, tofu, and mayonnaise that's so rich and flavorful, you won't miss the cheese one bit. Rosemary and Garlic Focaccia (page 46) makes a great accompaniment to this dish.

1 (8-OUNCE) BOX LARGE GLUTEN-FREE PASTA SHELLS

¼ POUND GROUND PORK SAUSAGE

2 CUPS CHOPPED FRESH SPINACH

1 (14-OUNCE) PACKAGE SOFT TOFU, DRAINED

1 EGG, LIGHTLY BEATEN

2 TABLESPOONS MAYONNAISE

2 TABLESPOONS CHOPPED FLAT-LEAF PARSLEY, PLUS MORE FOR GARNISH (OPTIONAL)

SALT

FRESHLY GROUND BLACK PEPPER

2 CUPS TOMATO SAUCE

2½ TABLESPOONS ALMOND FLOUR

1. Bring a large pot of water to boil over medium-high heat. Add the shells, bring the water back to a simmer, decrease the heat to medium-low, and cook for 6 minutes, or until the shells soften but are still firm. Drain and set aside to cool.

2. Preheat the oven to 350°F.

3. In a skillet over medium heat, cook the sausage for 2 to 3 minutes, until it begins to brown.

4. Stir in the chopped spinach and cook for 2 minutes, then remove the sausage mixture from the heat and let it cool for several minutes.

5. In a medium bowl, stir together the tofu, egg, mayonnaise, parsley, and cooled sausage mixture. Season with salt and pepper.

6. Spread about ¾ cup of the tomato sauce in the bottom of a large baking dish. Arrange the partially cooked shells in the dish on top of the sauce.

continued ▶

Dairy-Free Stuffed Pasta Shells *continued*

7. Spoon the tofu mixture into the shells, then pour the remaining sauce over them.

8. Sprinkle the shells with almond flour and additional parsley (if using).

9. Cover the shells with foil and bake them for 15 minutes, or until the shells are tender and the filling is hot.

10. Let the stuffed shells rest for 5 minutes before serving hot.

NUTRITIONAL INFORMATION PER SERVING: CALORIES 509 TOTAL FAT 22.7G SATURATED FAT 3.9G
TRANS FAT 0.0G SODIUM 993MG TOTAL CARBOHYDRATES 57.4G SUGARS 7.7G PROTEIN 21.8G

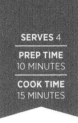
Lemon-Garlic Rotini with Spinach

This simple pasta dish uses brown rice rotini, but you could substitute any gluten-free pasta you like. Flavored with lemon and garlic and lightened up with tender spinach, it makes a lovely light supper. If you aren't avoiding dairy, sprinkle on a bit of freshly grated Parmesan.

Ingredient tip If you don't have fresh spinach, use thawed frozen spinach. Just be sure to squeeze out the excess moisture before adding it to the pasta.

12 OUNCES BROWN RICE ROTINI

1 TABLESPOON EXTRA-VIRGIN
     OLIVE OIL

1 TABLESPOON MINCED GARLIC

1 ONION, CHOPPED

2 TABLESPOONS FRESHLY SQUEEZED
     LEMON JUICE

4 CUPS GENTLY PACKED FRESH
     BABY SPINACH

1. Bring a large pot of salted water to a boil over medium-high heat. Add the rotini, bring the water back to a simmer, reduce the heat to medium, and cook according to the directions on the box until the rotini are al dente. Drain the pasta and set it aside.

2. Heat the olive oil in a large skillet over medium heat. Add the garlic and cook for 1 minute.

3. Stir in the onion and cook for 3 to 5 minutes, until tender.

4. Add the drained rotini and toss to coat the rotini with oil, then stir in the lemon juice.

5. Stir in the spinach and cook for 2 minutes, or until the spinach is just wilted. Serve hot.

NUTRITIONAL INFORMATION PER SERVING: CALORIES 337 TOTAL FAT 4.6G SATURATED FAT 0.6G
TRANS FAT 0.0G SODIUM 33MG TOTAL CARBOHYDRATES 67.2G SUGARS 6.0G PROTEIN 7.2G

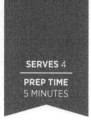

Ginger-Lime Soba Noodles

Soba noodles are Japanese noodles made from buckwheat flour. Despite its name, buckwheat is not a type of wheat and it does not contain gluten. With a nutty flavor and firm bite, soba noodles are delicious in hot dishes, and they work well chilled in salads.

Ingredient tip Although buckwheat is naturally gluten-free, many brands of soba noodles include some wheat as well. Be sure to read the label and choose a brand that is truly gluten-free. Eden Foods makes good wheat-free soba noodles.

3 TABLESPOONS GRATED FRESH GINGER

ZEST AND FRESHLY SQUEEZED JUICE OF 1 LIME

3 TABLESPOONS UNSEASONED RICE WINE VINEGAR

½ TEASPOON SALT

¼ TEASPOON FRESHLY GROUND BLACK PEPPER

½ CUP EXTRA-VIRGIN OLIVE OIL

8 OUNCES DRIED SOBA NOODLES, COOKED ACCORDING TO PACKAGE DIRECTIONS

1 CUP COOKED, SHELLED EDAMAME

½ CUP THINLY SLICED SCALLIONS, PLUS MORE FOR GARNISH

½ CUP CHOPPED ROASTED PEANUTS, PLUS MORE FOR GARNISH

1. In a medium bowl, combine the ginger, lime zest and juice, vinegar, salt, and pepper. While whisking, add the olive oil in a thin stream and continue whisking until the mixture is fully emulsified.

2. In a large bowl, combine the cooked noodles, dressing, edamame, scallions, and peanuts, and toss to combine.

3. Serve the noodles warm or chilled, garnished with additional scallions and peanuts.

NUTRITIONAL INFORMATION PER SERVING: CALORIES 594 TOTAL FAT 36.3G SATURATED FAT 5.0G TRANS FAT 0.0G SODIUM 876MG TOTAL CARBOHYDRATES 57.2G SUGARS 1.6G PROTEIN 17.8G

Cauliflower Crust Pizza with Red Onions, Zucchini, and Mozzarella

SERVES 4

PREP TIME
10 MINUTES

COOK TIME
45 MINUTES

This grain-free pizza uses a crust made out of cauliflower. Topped with a quick tomato sauce, vegetable toppings, and cheese, it will satisfy your pizza craving. Feel free to experiment with whatever toppings you like. The instructions may seem long, but rest assured, the whole thing is quick and easy to make.

Ingredient tip If you avoid dairy as well as gluten, use a dairy-free cheese, such as Daiya, instead of the mozzarella. Or you can make your own cashew "cheese." Soak a cup of raw cashews overnight, then drain them and process them in a blender or food processor along with 2 teaspoons of freshly squeezed lemon juice, ½ teaspoon of salt, and ¼ cup of water. Drizzle the cashew cheese onto the pizza before or after cooking.

FOR THE CRUST

1 HEAD CAULIFLOWER, STEM TRIMMED
    AND CUT INTO SMALL FLORETS

2 TABLESPOONS ALMOND FLOUR

1 TABLESPOON COCONUT OIL

½ TEASPOON DRIED BASIL

½ TEASPOON DRIED OREGANO

¼ TEASPOON SALT

1 EGG, LIGHTLY BEATEN

NONSTICK COOKING SPRAY

FOR THE SAUCE

2 TABLESPOONS COCONUT OIL

¼ ONION, DICED

3 GARLIC CLOVES, MINCED

1 (28-OUNCE) CAN DICED TOMATOES

1 TABLESPOON MINCED FRESH BASIL

1½ TEASPOONS SALT

½ TEASPOON FRESHLY GROUND
    BLACK PEPPER

FOR THE TOPPINGS

1 CUP SHREDDED MOZZARELLA
    CHEESE

½ RED ONION, THINLY SLICED

1 ZUCCHINI, THINLY SLICED

To make the crust

1. Place a pizza stone or baking sheet in the oven and preheat it to 450°F.

2. Fill a steamer pot with a couple of inches of water and bring to a boil.

continued ▶

3. Place the cauliflower in a food processor and pulse until it is in fine crumbs and looks a bit like snow. Transfer the cauliflower to a steamer basket and steam it over the boiling water for about 5 minutes.

4. Let the cauliflower cool, then transfer it to a clean dish towel and squeeze as much water out of it as you can.

5. In a medium bowl, combine the cooked and drained cauliflower with the almond flour, coconut oil, basil, oregano, and salt. Mix well. Add the egg and mix well.

6. Place a piece of parchment paper on the counter and spray it with nonstick cooking spray. Turn the dough out onto the prepared parchment paper and, using your hands, pat it out into a 10-inch round pizza crust.

7. Using the parchment paper, transfer the crust onto the heated pizza stone or baking sheet; discard the paper. Bake until the crust begins to turn golden, about 15 minutes. Remove the crust from the oven.

To make the sauce

1. While the crust is in the oven, make the sauce. Heat the coconut oil in a medium saucepan over medium-high heat. Add the onion and garlic and cook, stirring, until they soften, about 5 minutes.

2. Stir in the tomatoes, basil, salt, and pepper, and bring the mixture to a boil. Reduce the heat to medium-low, cover, and simmer for 10 minutes.

To make the pizza

1. Spoon several scoops of sauce onto the pizza crust and spread it in an even layer with the back of the spoon all the way to the edges of the crust.

2. Sprinkle the mozzarella cheese evenly over the sauce. Arrange the red onion and zucchini on top.

3. Bake the pizza for about 15 minutes, until the cheese is bubbly and the vegetables are beginning to brown.

4. Remove the pizza from the oven, cut it into wedges, and serve immediately.

NUTRITIONAL INFORMATION PER SERVING: CALORIES 338 TOTAL FAT 24.0G SATURATED FAT 12.8G
TRANS FAT; 0.0G SODIUM 1,245MG TOTAL CARBOHYDRATES 19.9G SUGARS 9.1G PROTEIN 16.4G

Spinach-Onion Frittata

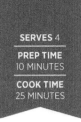

SERVES 4

PREP TIME
10 MINUTES

COOK TIME
25 MINUTES

Frittatas are a great way to serve eggs for a crowd. They are full of flavor, easy to make, and best of all, they are delicious either warm from the oven or at room temperature, so you can even make them ahead. This savory version is flavored with onions and spinach, but feel free to experiment with other vegetables, such as chard, kale, leeks, or shallots, and add other ingredients such as fresh herbs or shredded cheese, if you like.

Time-saving tip A frittata is incredibly forgiving. To save time, you can cook up a double batch and store it in the freezer. Defrost it in the refrigerator overnight and then bring it to room temperature by setting it on the countertop for 30 minutes before serving.

9 EGGS

2 TABLESPOONS FAT-FREE MILK

1 TEASPOON SALT

3 TABLESPOONS FRESHLY GRATED
    PARMESAN CHEESE

1 TABLESPOON EXTRA-VIRGIN
    OLIVE OIL

1 CUP DICED YELLOW ONION

4 CUPS CHOPPED FRESH SPINACH

1 GARLIC CLOVE, MINCED

1. Preheat the oven to 400°F.

2. In a medium bowl, beat the eggs until they are thoroughly combined. Whisk in the milk, salt, and Parmesan cheese. Set aside.

3. Heat the olive oil in a medium ovenproof skillet over medium heat. Add the onion and cook, stirring frequently, for 4 minutes, or until soft.

4. Stir in the spinach and garlic and cook for 1 minute more, stirring often.

5. Spread the vegetable mixture evenly in the skillet and pour the egg mixture over it.

6. Let the frittata cook undisturbed for 5 minutes, until halfway set, then transfer the skillet, uncovered, to the oven.

7. Bake the frittata for 8 to 12 minutes, until it is puffed and golden brown on top.

8. Remove the frittata from the oven and let it sit for 5 minutes.

9. To serve, cut it into wedges. Serve the frittata hot or at room temperature.

NUTRITIONAL INFORMATION PER SERVING: CALORIES 262   TOTAL FAT 18.0G   SATURATED FAT 6.6G
TRANS FAT 0.0G   SODIUM 943MG   TOTAL CARBOHYDRATES 5.9G   SUGARS 2.5G   PROTEIN 20.6G

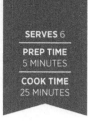

Garden Vegetable Frittata with Basil

Like a quiche without the crust, frittata is a quick, satisfying, and healthy meal. Just add a crisp green salad with vinaigrette, and you're good to go. This version combines broccoli, chard, and red onion, but you can mix it up with whatever you have on hand. Try zucchini, corn, and cherry tomatoes in the summertime or leeks, peas, and baby spinach in the spring.

3 TABLESPOONS UNSALTED BUTTER

1 RED ONION, DICED

1 HEAD BROCCOLI, CUT INTO
    BITE-SIZE PIECES

1 POUND CHARD, STURDY RIBS
    DISCARDED, LEAVES JULIENNED

8 EGGS

¾ CUP HALF-AND-HALF OR
    WHOLE MILK

½ TEASPOON SALT

¼ TEASPOON FRESHLY GROUND
    BLACK PEPPER

1½ CUPS SHREDDED
    JARLSBERG CHEESE

¼ CUP CHOPPED FRESH BASIL

¼ CUP FRESHLY GRATED
    PARMESAN CHEESE

1. Melt the butter in a large nonstick skillet set over medium-high heat. Add the onion and broccoli and cook, stirring frequently, until the onions are translucent, about 5 minutes.

2. Add the chard and cook another 2 or 3 minutes, until the chard is tender.

3. In a medium bowl, whisk together the eggs, half-and-half, salt, and pepper until well blended. Stir in the shredded Jarlsberg cheese and basil. Pour the mixture over the vegetables. Sprinkle the Parmesan cheese over the top.

4. Reduce the heat to low, cover the pan, and cook for about 20 minutes, until the eggs are completely set and the frittata begins to puff up. Serve immediately.

NUTRITIONAL INFORMATION PER SERVING: CALORIES 365 TOTAL FAT 28.0G SATURATED FAT 15.6G TRANS FAT 0.0G SODIUM 822MG TOTAL CARBOHYDRATES 7.8G SUGARS 2.4G PROTEIN 22.5G

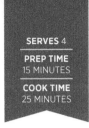
Black Bean and Pumpkin Enchiladas with Salsa

A zesty sauce, thickened with arrowroot starch, blankets these hearty vegetarian enchiladas filled with protein-rich black beans and pumpkin purée. Topped with a bit of melted cheese and served alongside a crisp green salad, this is an easy and satisfying vegetarian meal.

Time-saving tip Filling and rolling each tortilla individually is the most time-consuming part of this recipe. To speed things up, make a stacked enchilada casserole instead. Cover the bottom of the baking dish with salsa, then a layer of tortillas (cut them into pieces to cover the dish in a single layer). Next add a layer of sauce, a layer of pumpkin purée, a layer of the bean mixture, then another layer of tortillas. Repeat, layering salsa, pumpkin purée, bean mixture, and then top with a final layer of tortillas, the remaining salsa, and the cheese.

FOR THE SALSA VERDE

1 CUP GLUTEN-FREE
    VEGETABLE BROTH

1 TABLESPOON ARROWROOT STARCH
    DISSOLVED IN 1 TABLESPOON
    COLD WATER

1 (8-OUNCE) CAN ROASTED GREEN
    CHILES, CHOPPED

3 GARLIC CLOVES, MINCED

1 TEASPOON GROUND CUMIN

1 TEASPOON CHILI POWDER

FOR THE ENCHILADAS

EXTRA-VIRGIN OLIVE OIL OR
    VEGETABLE OIL, FOR PREPARING
    THE BAKING PAN

1 (15-OUNCE) CAN BLACK BEANS,
    DRAINED AND RINSED

1 (4-OUNCE) CAN ROASTED GREEN
    CHILES, CHOPPED

3 GARLIC CLOVES, MINCED

FRESHLY SQUEEZED JUICE OF 1 LIME

1 (15-OUNCE) CAN PUMPKIN PURÉE

½ TEASPOON GROUND CUMIN

½ TEASPOON CHILI POWDER

SALT

FRESHLY GROUND BLACK PEPPER

8 WHITE OR YELLOW CORN TORTILLAS

SHREDDED MONTEREY JACK CHEESE

2 TABLESPOONS CHOPPED FRESH
    CILANTRO, FOR GARNISH

continued ▶

To make the salsa verde

1. In a small saucepan, mix together the vegetable broth, arrowroot mixture, green chiles, garlic, cumin, and chili powder.

2. Place the pan over medium-high heat and bring the mixture almost to a boil. Reduce the heat and simmer until the sauce thickens, about 5 minutes.

To make the enchiladas

1. Preheat the oven to 350°F.

2. Lightly oil a 9-by-13-inch baking dish.

3. In a medium bowl, stir together the beans, chiles, garlic, and lime juice.

4. In another medium bowl, stir together the pumpkin purée, cumin, and chili powder. Season with salt and pepper.

5. Spoon several tablespoons of the salsa into the prepared baking dish and spread it out with the back of the spoon.

6. If using a gas stove, heat each tortilla briefly on both sides over the open flame before filling it. If using an electric stove, heat a skillet over medium-high heat and heat the tortillas, one at a time, for 30 seconds or so on each side.

7. To fill the enchiladas, lay a hot tortilla in the sauce in the baking dish and turn it over to coat it with the salsa. Dollop a couple of tablespoons of the pumpkin mixture in a line down the center of the tortilla. Top with a similar amount of the black bean mixture. Roll the tortilla up around the filling and place it at one end of the baking dish, seam side down. Repeat with the remaining tortillas.

8. When all of the tortillas are filled and placed in the baking dish, spoon the remaining salsa over the top. Sprinkle with the Monterey Jack cheese.

9. Bake the enchiladas for about 20 minutes, until the sauce and cheese are bubbling and the cheese begins to brown.

10. Serve hot, garnished with cilantro.

NUTRITIONAL INFORMATION PER SERVING: CALORIES 594 TOTAL FAT 9.3G SATURATED FAT 1.4G
TRANS FAT 0.4G SODIUM 174MG TOTAL CARBOHYDRATES 110.7G SUGARS 12.4G PROTEIN 29.2G

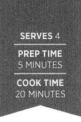
Masala-Curried Chickpeas

Chickpeas are a delicious and inexpensive protein source. Keep a few cans around, and you'll always be able to whip up a tasty and satisfying meal. Garam masala is an Indian spice mix. If you like your curry spicy, double the chiles or add a bit of cayenne pepper. Serve this saucy dish over rice for a complete protein.

Ingredient tip Fresh ginger keeps well in the freezer. If you have extra, peel it and stash it in a resealable bag in your freezer. Frozen ginger is also much easier to grate than fresh.

1 TABLESPOON UNSALTED BUTTER
    OR GHEE
1 YELLOW ONION, DICED
1 TABLESPOON GARAM MASALA
1 TABLESPOON TOMATO PASTE
2 TEASPOONS GRATED FRESH GINGER
1 SERRANO CHILE, MINCED
½ TEASPOON SALT

2 (15-OUNCE) CANS CHICKPEAS,
    DRAINED AND RINSED
1 (28-OUNCE) CAN CRUSHED
    TOMATOES
½ CUP LOW-FAT PLAIN GREEK YOGURT
¼ CUP CHOPPED FRESH CILANTRO,
    FOR GARNISH

1. Melt the butter in a large skillet over medium heat. Add the onion and cook, stirring frequently, until it softens, about 5 minutes.

2. Stir in the garam masala, tomato paste, ginger, chile, and salt, and cook, stirring, for about 1 minute.

3. Add the chickpeas and tomatoes, increase the heat to high, and bring the mixture to a boil.

4. Lower the heat and simmer, uncovered, stirring occasionally, for 15 minutes. Remove the pan from the heat.

5. Just before serving, stir in the yogurt.

6. Serve the chickpeas over steamed white or brown rice, garnished with cilantro.

NUTRITIONAL INFORMATION PER SERVING: CALORIES 617   TOTAL FAT 11.1G   SATURATED FAT 2.5G
SODIUM 512MG   TOTAL CARBOHYDRATES 99.7G   SUGARS 24.6G   PROTEIN 33.7G

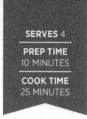

Smoky Lentils with Vegetables

Lentils are quick to cook, and with their earthy flavor and high nutrition content, they make a fantastic vegetarian meal. Chopped smoked almonds add crunch and an unexpected hint of smoky flavor.

Ingredient tip Brown lentils have an earthy flavor and cook quickly, in about 20 minutes. With a sweet, nutty flavor, red lentils are a beautiful alternative to brown, but they take a bit longer to cook, about 30 minutes. Green lentils, which have a stronger flavor with a hint of pepper, take the longest to cook, about 45 minutes.

1 TABLESPOON SESAME OIL

2½ TEASPOONS WHOLE CUMIN SEEDS

1 CARROT, CHOPPED

1 CELERY STALK, CHOPPED

1 LEEK, TRIMMED AND CHOPPED

3 GARLIC CLOVES, MINCED

3 CUPS GLUTEN-FREE
    VEGETABLE BROTH

1 CUP BROWN LENTILS, DRAINED
    AND RINSED

SALT

FRESHLY GROUND BLACK PEPPER

¾ CUP UNSALTED SMOKED ALMONDS,
    COARSELY CHOPPED, FOR GARNISH

½ CUP PLAIN GREEK YOGURT,
    FOR GARNISH

1. Heat the sesame oil in a stockpot set over low heat. Add the cumin seeds and cook, stirring, until fragrant, about 1 minute.

2. Increase the heat to high and add the carrot, celery, leek, and garlic. Cook, stirring, until the vegetables begin to soften, about 3 minutes.

3. Add the vegetable broth and lentils and lower the heat. Simmer, uncovered, until the lentils are tender, about 20 minutes.

4. Season with salt and pepper.

5. Serve hot, garnished with the almonds and yogurt.

NUTRITIONAL INFORMATION PER SERVING: CALORIES 307 TOTAL FAT 9.3G SATURATED FAT 0.9G
TRANS FAT 0.0G **SODIUM** 97MG **TOTAL CARBOHYDRATES** 40.3G **SUGARS** 7.7G **PROTEIN** 18.6G

NOTES

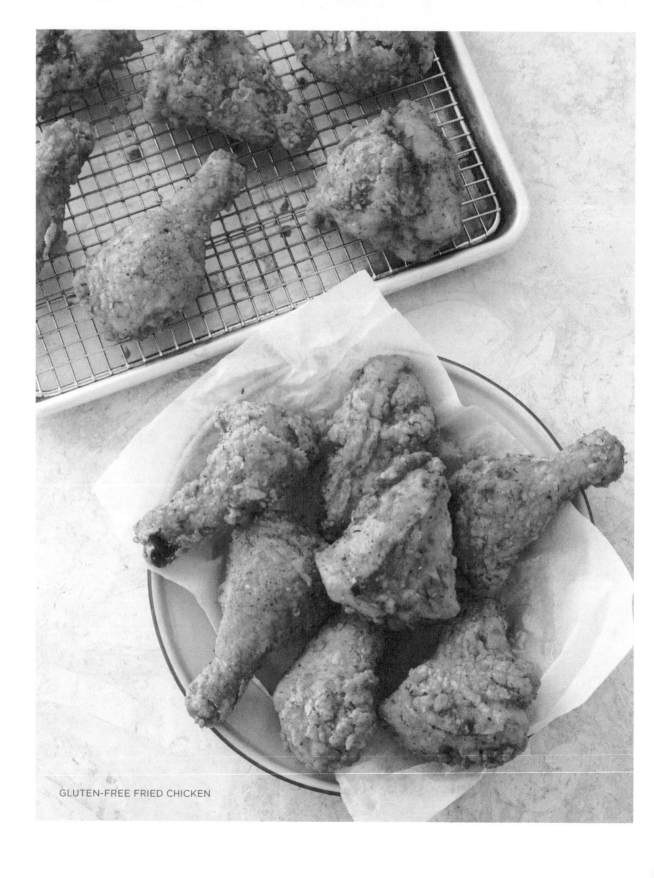

GLUTEN-FREE FRIED CHICKEN

10

Fish, Seafood, and Meat Entrées

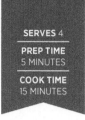

Honey-Lemon Baked Halibut

Halibut is a firm white fish with a mild flavor that pairs well with just about anything. Here, meaty halibut fillets are brushed with honey for a subtly sweet flavor and topped with lemon—the perfect way to serve fish.

4 (6-OUNCE) HALIBUT FILLETS
SALT
FRESHLY GROUND BLACK PEPPER
1 TABLESPOON HONEY

2 TEASPOONS EXTRA-VIRGIN
OLIVE OIL
1 LEMON, CUT INTO THIN SLICES

1. Preheat the oven to 350°F.

2. Rinse the fillets well and pat them dry with paper towels. Season the fillets with salt and pepper.

3. Arrange the fillets in a roasting pan.

4. In a small bowl, whisk together the honey and olive oil.

5. Brush the fillets with the honey-oil mixture, then cover them with the lemon slices.

6. Bake the fillets for 12 to 15 minutes, until the flesh of the fish flakes easily with a fork.

7. Serve the halibut hot with extra lemon slices.

NUTRITIONAL INFORMATION PER SERVING: CALORIES 274 TOTAL FAT 7.3G SATURATED FAT 1.0G
TRANS FAT 0.0G SODIUM 156MG TOTAL CARBOHYDRATES 4.3G SUGARS 4.3G PROTEIN 45.4G

Coconut-Crusted Haddock

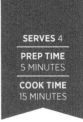
Haddock gets a delicious coating of flaked coconut and coconut flour that makes for a crunchy finish when baked in the oven. This dish provides the fried fish experience with zero gluten, far less fat, and fewer calories than traditional fish and chips.

4 (6-OUNCE) HADDOCK FILLETS
SALT
FRESHLY GROUND BLACK PEPPER

4 TABLESPOONS UNSWEETENED
FLAKED COCONUT
1 TABLESPOON COCONUT FLOUR
¼ TEASPOON DRIED OREGANO

1. Preheat the oven to 350°F.

2. Rinse the fillets and pat them dry with paper towels. Season the fillets with salt and pepper.

3. Arrange the fillets on a roasting pan.

4. In a small bowl, combine the coconut, coconut flour, and oregano.

5. Sprinkle the mixture liberally over the fillets.

6. Bake the fillets for 12 to 15 minutes, until the flesh of the fish flakes easily with a fork.

7. Serve hot.

NUTRITIONAL INFORMATION PER SERVING: **CALORIES** 216 **TOTAL FAT** 3.4G **SATURATED FAT** 1.8G **TRANS FAT** 0.0G **SODIUM** 192MG **TOTAL CARBOHYDRATES** 1.8G **SUGARS** 0.0G **PROTEIN** 41.7G

Maple-Glazed Tuna Steaks

Tuna steaks are thick cuts that are best prepared by searing the outside and leaving the center still pink and succulent. These are delicious brushed with a sweet-savory maple glaze. Serve this light and healthy entrée with a crisp green salad and quinoa or brown rice on the side.

Cooking tip If you are uncomfortable eating very rare fish, substitute an oilier type, like salmon, and cook it all the way through.

2 TABLESPOONS PURE MAPLE SYRUP

2 TABLESPOONS FRESHLY SQUEEZED
    LIME JUICE

PINCH MUSTARD POWDER

4 TABLESPOONS EXTRA-VIRGIN
    OLIVE OIL

4 (6-OUNCE) SUSHI-GRADE
    TUNA STEAKS

SALT

FRESHLY GROUND BLACK PEPPER

1. In a small bowl, whisk together the maple syrup, lime juice, and mustard powder with 1 tablespoon of olive oil.

2. Season the tuna steaks with salt and pepper.

3. Heat the remaining 3 tablespoons of olive oil in a heavy skillet over high heat.

4. Add the tuna and sear the steaks for 30 to 45 seconds on each side. The outside of the tuna should be opaque but the center still pink.

5. Transfer the steaks to a serving plate and brush them with the maple-lime glaze. Serve hot.

NUTRITIONAL INFORMATION PER SERVING: CALORIES 377   TOTAL FAT 17.5G   SATURATED FAT 2.0G
TRANS FAT 0.0G   SODIUM 40MG   TOTAL CARBOHYDRATES 8.6G   SUGARS 6.3G   PROTEIN 47.7G

Simple Salmon Burgers

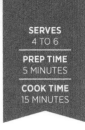

SERVES
4 TO 6

PREP TIME
5 MINUTES

COOK TIME
15 MINUTES

These salmon burgers are seasoned with Japanese ume plum vinegar, a strong, salty brew infused with the flavor of Japanese umeboshi plums. Serve the burgers on a bed of lettuce with a drizzle of lemon juice or, if you prefer, in a gluten-free burger bun dressed with mayonnaise and topped with greens.

Ingredient tip Ume plum vinegar, also called umeboshi vinegar, is a little fruity and quite salty. If you can't find it, substitute red wine vinegar mixed with a little salt or gluten-free soy sauce.

1 POUND SKINLESS SALMON FILLETS

1 TABLESPOON SESAME OIL

1 TABLESPOON UME PLUM VINEGAR

1 TEASPOON MINCED GARLIC

1 TEASPOON GRATED FRESH GINGER

¼ CUP DICED RED ONION

2 EGGS, LIGHTLY BEATEN

1 TABLESPOON COCONUT FLOUR

1 TABLESPOON EXTRA-VIRGIN OLIVE OIL

1. Rinse the salmon well and pat it dry with paper towels. Chop it into small cubes.

2. In a medium bowl, with a wooden spoon or your hands, mix together the chopped salmon, sesame oil, vinegar, garlic, ginger, onion, and eggs.

3. Add the coconut flour and mix well.

4. Shape the mixture into patties using a ¼-cup measure.

5. Heat the olive oil in a heavy medium skillet over medium-high heat.

6. Add the patties to the skillet and cook them for 4 to 6 minutes on each side, until they are lightly browned. Cook the patties in batches to avoid crowding, if necessary.

7. Drain the patties on a paper towel-lined plate. Serve hot.

NUTRITIONAL INFORMATION PER SERVING: CALORIES 306   TOTAL FAT 21.3G   SATURATED FAT 4.2G
TRANS FAT 0.0G   SODIUM 888MG   TOTAL CARBOHYDRATES 2.4G   SUGARS 0.6G   PROTEIN 25.3G

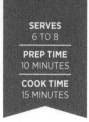

SERVES
6 TO 8

PREP TIME
10 MINUTES

COOK TIME
15 MINUTES

Bacon-Wrapped Sea Scallops

On their own, sea scallops are sweet, tender, and delicious. Wrapped in bacon and broiled, they are the food of gods. This recipe makes an easy but impressive main dish. To serve it as an appetizer, use smaller bay scallops and cut the bacon to fit.

1½ POUNDS SEA SCALLOPS

SALT

FRESHLY GROUND BLACK PEPPER

¾ POUND THINLY SLICED BACON

1. Rinse the scallops well in cool water and pat dry. Season them with salt and pepper.

2. Preheat the broiler to high.

3. Wrap each scallop with a slice of bacon and spear it with a toothpick to secure the bacon.

4. Arrange the scallops on a broiler pan and cook them for 10 to 15 minutes, until the bacon is cooked through, turning once halfway through.

5. Drain the scallops on paper towels and serve hot.

NUTRITIONAL INFORMATION PER SERVING: CALORIES 407   TOTAL FAT 24.6G   SATURATED FAT 7.9G
TRANS FAT 0.0G   SODIUM 1,519MG   TOTAL CARBOHYDRATES 3.5G   SUGARS 0.0G   PROTEIN 40.0G

Garlic-Lime Grilled Shrimp

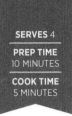

SERVES 4

PREP TIME
10 MINUTES

COOK TIME
5 MINUTES

This grilled shrimp takes only a few minutes to prepare and a few more to cook, making it the perfect recipe for your next backyard barbecue. Serve them with gluten-free corn tortillas, salsa, guacamole, and other toppings for a make-your-own shrimp taco bar.

EXTRA-VIRGIN OLIVE OIL, FOR
    THE GRILL
2 POUNDS SHRIMP, PEELED AND
    DEVEINED
1 TABLESPOON MINCED GARLIC
SALT

FRESHLY GROUND BLACK PEPPER
2 TABLESPOONS CHOPPED FRESH
    CILANTRO
1 TABLESPOON FRESHLY SQUEEZED
    LIME JUICE
3 LIMES, CUT INTO THIN SLICES

1. Soak the wooden skewers in water for 1 hour before using.

2. Heat a grill or grill pan to medium heat and brush the grate with olive oil or heat the broiler to high.

3. Place the shrimp in a medium bowl. Sprinkle with garlic, season with salt and pepper, and then toss with cilantro and lime juice.

4. Thread the shrimp onto the skewers, alternating with a slice of lime between each shrimp.

5. Grill or broil the skewers for 1 to 2 minutes on each side, until the shrimp are just cooked through.

6. Serve the shrimp hot with extra lime slices for garnish.

NUTRITIONAL INFORMATION PER SERVING: **CALORIES** 318 **TOTAL FAT** 7.4G **SATURATED FAT** 1.7G
TRANS FAT 0.0G **SODIUM** 594MG **TOTAL CARBOHYDRATES** 9.5G **SUGARS** 0.9G **PROTEIN** 52.1G

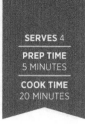

Gluten-Free Fried Chicken

Even though there is so much variety in gluten-free cooking and so many great products available, many people find they really miss the old classics when they go gluten-free. Here is a recipe that turns out such crispy, delicious fried chicken that it will make you forget all about gluten.

Cooking tip Don't crowd the chicken while it's frying. If necessary, cook it in batches.

1 QUART BUTTERMILK

1 TABLESPOON PAPRIKA

2 TEASPOONS GARLIC POWDER

2 TEASPOONS ONION POWDER

2½ TEASPOONS SALT, DIVIDED

1½ TEASPOONS FRESHLY GROUND
    BLACK PEPPER, DIVIDED

2 CHICKEN BREASTS, EACH CUT IN HALF

2 CHICKEN THIGHS

2 CHICKEN LEGS

2 CHICKEN WINGS

1½ CUPS GLUTEN-FREE
    ALL-PURPOSE FLOUR

1 TABLESPOON SMOKED PAPRIKA

4 CUPS CANOLA OIL

1. In a large bowl, combine the buttermilk, paprika, garlic power, onion powder, 1½ teaspoons of salt, and ½ teaspoon of pepper. Add the chicken and mix to coat all sides of the chicken.

2. In a shallow bowl, combine the flour, remaining 1 teaspoon of salt, remaining 1 teaspoon of pepper, and smoked paprika.

3. Pour the canola oil into a large skillet and heat it over medium-high heat.

4. When the oil is very hot (360°F), pull one piece of chicken at a time out of the buttermilk mixture, let the excess liquid run off, and dredge the chicken in the flour mixture. Place the chicken in the hot oil and repeat with the remaining chicken.

5. Cook the chicken until it is nicely browned and cooked through, about 20 minutes, turning it once during cooking.

6. Drain the chicken on paper towels and serve immediately.

NUTRITIONAL INFORMATION PER SERVING: CALORIES 825 TOTAL FAT 43.6G SATURATED FAT 10.6G TRANS FAT 0.0G SODIUM 2,020MG TOTAL CARBOHYDRATES 50.7G SUGARS 12.9G PROTEIN 55.6G

Maple-Lime Chicken

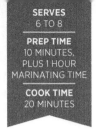

SERVES
6 TO 8

PREP TIME
10 MINUTES,
PLUS 1 HOUR
MARINATING TIME

COOK TIME
20 MINUTES

The flavors of maple and lime combine perfectly in this recipe to create a tender, juicy chicken breast in a sweet-savory glaze. Serve this chicken with rice or quinoa and a crisp green salad with feta cheese and nuts.

Ingredient tip If you are sensitive to soy as well as gluten, you can substitute coconut aminos for the soy sauce.

½ CUP PURE MAPLE SYRUP

¾ CUP FRESHLY SQUEEZED LIME JUICE

2 TABLESPOONS GLUTEN-FREE
    SOY SAUCE

8 BONELESS CHICKEN THIGHS

SALT

FRESHLY GROUND BLACK PEPPER

1 TABLESPOON EXTRA-VIRGIN
    OLIVE OIL

1. In a small bowl, whisk together the maple syrup, lime juice, and soy sauce.

2. Season the chicken with salt and pepper and place it in a shallow dish. Pour the marinade over the chicken and marinate it in the refrigerator for 1 hour.

3. Heat the olive oil in a large skillet over medium-high heat. Add the chicken (reserving the marinade) and cook for 2 minutes on each side, until browned.

4. Pour in the marinade, bring it to a simmer, and reduce the heat to low. Simmer the chicken, covered, for 15 minutes, or until it is cooked through.

5. Serve hot.

NUTRITIONAL INFORMATION PER SERVING: CALORIES 412 TOTAL FAT 25.1G SATURATED FAT 7.0G
TRANS FAT 0.0G SODIUM 470MG TOTAL CARBOHYDRATES 17.9G SUGARS 15.6G PROTEIN 27.3G

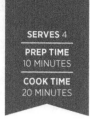
Skillet Chicken Parmesan

Chicken Parmesan is an Italian favorite that you may have thought you had to give up because of the breading. By substituting almond flour, this recipe earns back a prized spot on your table. This is a quicker prep that's all done on the stove top.

Cooking tip To keep the chicken super moist during cooking, spread each piece all over with a thin layer of mayonnaise before dipping it in the egg. It seems weird, but it's an old family secret that really does the trick.

4 BONELESS, SKINLESS CHICKEN
    BREAST HALVES
1 EGG
¼ CUP ALMOND FLOUR
1 TEASPOON ITALIAN
    SEASONING MIX
¼ TEASPOON SALT

2 TABLESPOONS EXTRA-VIRGIN
    OLIVE OIL
2 CUPS TOMATO SAUCE
½ CUP SHREDDED
    MOZZARELLA CHEESE
2 TABLESPOONS FRESHLY GRATED
    PARMESAN CHEESE

1. Place the chicken breast halves between 2 pieces of plastic wrap and gently pound them to about ¼-inch thick with a meat mallet.

2. In a shallow dish, beat the egg and set aside.

3. In another shallow dish, combine the almond flour, Italian seasoning, and salt.

4. Heat the olive oil in a large skillet over medium-high heat.

5. Dip the chicken pieces in the egg, then dredge them in the almond flour mixture to coat.

6. Place the chicken in the skillet and cook for 2 minutes on each side, until browned. Reduce the heat to medium and let the chicken cook for 5 to 10 minutes longer, until cooked through.

7. Pour the tomato sauce into the skillet and sprinkle the chicken with mozzarella cheese.

8. Reduce the heat to medium-low, cover, and let it cook for 3 to 5 minutes, until the cheese is melted.

9. Sprinkle the chicken with Parmesan cheese and serve hot.

NUTRITIONAL INFORMATION PER SERVING: CALORIES 480 TOTAL FAT 25.5G SATURATED FAT 7.9G
TRANS FAT 0.0G SODIUM 1,158MG TOTAL CARBOHYDRATES 8.5G SUGARS 5.4G PROTEIN 54.2G

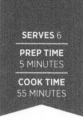
Rosemary Chicken with Vegetables

With cauliflower, carrots, and zucchini baked right along with the chicken, this one-dish dinner is an easy meal. Just throw the ingredients together and roast to perfection. If you're craving a carbohydrate to round out the meal, add a handful of quartered baby potatoes along with the other vegetables.

2 POUNDS BONE-IN CHICKEN
    DRUMSTICKS AND THIGHS

SALT

FRESHLY GROUND BLACK PEPPER

2 CUPS CAULIFLOWER FLORETS

1 CUP HALVED BABY CARROTS

1 YELLOW ONION, QUARTERED

1 ZUCCHINI, CUT INTO 1-INCH CHUNKS

2 TABLESPOONS DRIED ROSEMARY

¼ CUP GLUTEN-FREE CHICKEN BROTH

1. Preheat the oven to 400°F.

2. Season the chicken with salt and pepper and set aside.

3. In a 9-by-13-inch glass baking dish, combine the cauliflower, carrots, onion, and zucchini, and top with the chicken.

4. Sprinkle the chicken and vegetables with the dried rosemary and then drizzle them with the chicken broth.

5. Roast the chicken for 45 to 55 minutes, or until the chicken is cooked through and very tender.

6. Serve the chicken hot with the vegetables on the side.

NUTRITIONAL INFORMATION PER SERVING: CALORIES 381 TOTAL FAT 20.6G SATURATED FAT 5.7G TRANS FAT 0.0G SODIUM 184MG TOTAL CARBOHYDRATES 6.4G SUGARS 2.8G PROTEIN 40.6G

Herb-Roasted Chicken

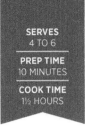

SERVES
4 TO 6

PREP TIME
10 MINUTES

COOK TIME
1½ HOURS

Though this recipe may take a little more time to cook than some of the others in this book, the preparation could not be simpler or quicker. And it's a wonderful option if you are feeding a crowd. By the way, you can save those chicken giblets in the freezer, and when you have a bagful, use them to make your own chicken soup.

Time-saving tip If your oven is large enough, save time by roasting two chickens at once. Eat one for supper tonight and save the other to use in sandwiches, salads, and casseroles throughout the week.

1 (2- TO 3-POUND) ROASTING CHICKEN

SALT

FRESHLY GROUND BLACK PEPPER

1 TABLESPOON CHOPPED
    FRESH THYME

1 TABLESPOON CHOPPED
    FRESH ROSEMARY

1 TEASPOON MINCED GARLIC

1. Preheat the oven to 425°F.

2. Remove the giblets bag from the cavity of the chicken and rinse the chicken inside and out with cool water. Pat it dry with paper towels.

3. Place the chicken in a roasting pan and season it liberally with salt and pepper.

4. In a small bowl, combine the thyme, rosemary, and garlic, and then rub the mixture into the skin of the chicken.

5. Tie the legs together with string and tuck the wings under the body of the chicken.

6. Roast the chicken for 1½ hours, or until the chicken's juices run clear.

7. Transfer the chicken to a cutting board and let it sit for 10 minutes before carving.

NUTRITIONAL INFORMATION PER SERVING: CALORIES 385   TOTAL FAT 15.2G   SATURATED FAT 4.2G
TRANS FAT 0.0G   SODIUM 210MG   TOTAL CARBOHYDRATES 1.2G   SUGARS 0.0G   PROTEIN 56.9G

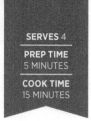
Chipotle Turkey Burgers

Ground turkey is a lean alternative to ground beef, and it makes a flavorful burger. Try these chipotle turkey burgers to taste for yourself. Serve them topped with cheese, salsa, and guacamole or the more traditional pickle slices and mustard—or any burger toppings you like.

Time-saving tip Uncooked turkey burgers freeze well. Mix up a double or triple batch, wrap the extras individually in plastic wrap, and freeze them for quick future meals. Simply defrost the burgers overnight in the refrigerator, then follow the cooking directions above.

1 POUND GROUND TURKEY

2 TABLESPOONS MINCED RED ONION

1 TABLESPOON ALMOND FLOUR

1 GARLIC CLOVE, MINCED

1 TEASPOON CHIPOTLE CHILI POWDER

1. Preheat the broiler to high.

2. In a medium bowl, combine the turkey, onion, flour, garlic, and chili powder, and mix well by hand.

3. Shape the mixture into 4 patties and place them on a broiler pan.

4. Broil the turkey burgers for 4 to 6 minutes on each side, until cooked through.

5. Serve the burgers hot on gluten-free burger buns with your favorite toppings.

NUTRITIONAL INFORMATION PER SERVING: CALORIES 267 **TOTAL FAT** 16.1G **SATURATED FAT** 2.3G
TRANS FAT 0.0G **SODIUM** 131MG **TOTAL CARBOHYDRATES** 2.6G **SUGARS** 0.5G **PROTEIN** 32.7G

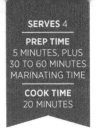

SERVES 4

PREP TIME
5 MINUTES, PLUS
30 TO 60 MINUTES
MARINATING TIME

COOK TIME
20 MINUTES

Rosemary Roasted Lamb Chops

Lamb is not only a great source of protein, but it is also rich in selenium and several B vitamins, including B3 and B12. Marinating the lamb chops in olive oil, garlic, and fresh herbs infuses them with intense flavor.

1 TABLESPOON MINCED GARLIC

1 TABLESPOON CHOPPED FRESH
    ROSEMARY

1 TABLESPOON CHOPPED
    FRESH THYME

2 TABLESPOONS EXTRA-VIRGIN
    OLIVE OIL, DIVIDED

8 (1¼-INCH-THICK) LAMB CHOPS

SALT

FRESHLY GROUND BLACK PEPPER

1. In a small bowl, combine the garlic, rosemary, thyme, and 1 tablespoon of olive oil.

2. Place the lamb chops in a shallow dish and season them with salt and pepper. Pour the marinade over the chops, turning to coat them.

3. Let the lamb chops marinate at room temperature for 30 to 60 minutes.

4. Preheat the oven to 400°F.

5. Heat the remaining 1 tablespoon of olive oil in a large skillet over high heat. Add the lamb chops and cook them for 2 to 3 minutes on each side, until browned.

6. Transfer the lamb chops to a roasting pan and roast them for 10 minutes for medium-rare.

7. Remove the chops to a platter and let them stand for 5 minutes before serving.

NUTRITIONAL INFORMATION PER SERVING: **CALORIES** 558 **TOTAL FA:T** 45.0G **SATURATED FAT** 20.3G
TRANS FAT 0.0G **SODIUM;** 40MG **TOTAL CARBOHYDRATES** 1.7G **SUGARS** 0.0G **PROTEIN** 37.2G

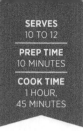

SERVES
10 TO 12

PREP TIME
10 MINUTES

COOK TIME
1 HOUR,
45 MINUTES

Pineapple-Glazed Ham

This pineapple-glazed ham is a great dish to serve at your next holiday gathering or dinner party. It is easy to prepare and serves a crowd. But don't worry if you don't have a huge crowd to serve. The leftovers are fantastic in sandwiches (try the Leftover Holiday Ham Sandwiches with Hot-Sweet Mustard on Pretzel Rolls, page 51).

1 (2½- TO 3-POUND) FULLY COOKED
    BONE-IN HAM

¾ CUP PINEAPPLE JUICE

1 (10-OUNCE) JAR PINEAPPLE
    PRESERVES

2 (8-OUNCE) CANS SLICED PINEAPPLE

1. Preheat the oven to 325°F.

2. Place the ham on a roasting rack in a roasting pan.

3. Use a sharp knife to make ½-inch-deep scores in the surface of the ham.

4. Pour the pineapple juice over the ham, then cover it with foil and bake it for 1 hour and 15 minutes.

5. Uncover the ham and brush it with the juices from the roasting pan as well as the pineapple preserves.

6. Spear pineapple slices with wooden toothpicks and stick them onto the ham.

7. Bake the ham for another 25 to 30 minutes, or until it is heated through. Slice to serve.

NUTRITIONAL INFORMATION PER SERVING: CALORIES 322 TOTAL FAT 14.7G SATURATED FAT 4.9G TRANS FAT 0.0G SODIUM 1,192MG TOTAL CARBOHYDRATES 26.8G SUGARS 23.4G PROTEIN 22.2G

Bacon-Wrapped Pork Chops

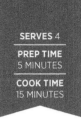

SERVES 4

PREP TIME
5 MINUTES

COOK TIME
15 MINUTES

Pork and bacon are two staples of the meat lover's diet, and in this recipe they come together in one perfect dish. Besides being delicious, the bacon also keeps the meat from becoming dry, which is always a risk with lean pork cuts such as loin.

Cooking tip Lean cuts of pork, like the loin, can dry out during cooking. Brining them ahead of time—soaking them in a saltwater solution—ensures they stay moist and tender. To brine pork chops, combine ¼ cup of salt with 4 cups of water. Place the chops in the solution and refrigerate them for 30 minutes to 2 hours. Rinse and pat the chops dry before cooking.

4 (6-OUNCE) BONELESS PORK
   LOIN CHOPS

SALT

FRESHLY GROUND BLACK PEPPER

4 THICK SLICES BACON

1. Preheat the broiler to high.

2. Pat the pork chops dry with a paper towel and season them with salt and pepper.

3. Wrap each chop with a slice of bacon and secure the bacon in place with a wooden toothpick.

4. Place the chops on a broiler pan and broil them for 6 minutes, then turn the chops over.

5. Broil the chops for another 5 to 6 minutes, until they are cooked to an internal temperature of at least 145°F.

6. Let the chops rest for 3 minutes before serving.

NUTRITIONAL INFORMATION PER SERVING: CALORIES 346   TOTAL FAT 13.9G   SATURATED FAT 4.7G
TRANS FAT 0.1G   SODIUM 575MG   TOTAL CARBOHYDRATES 0.3G   SUGARS 0.0G   PROTEIN 51.6G

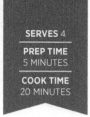

Bourbon-Glazed Pork Chops

A sweet-savory bourbon glaze makes this dish extra special. Serve the chops along-side mashed or roasted potatoes and sautéed greens for a meal that's worthy of Sunday dinner but can be easily prepared on a busy weeknight.

NONSTICK COOKING SPRAY

1 TABLESPOON EXTRA-VIRGIN
    OLIVE OIL

½ CUP CHOPPED PECANS

¾ CUP GLUTEN-FREE CHICKEN BROTH

¼ CUP BOURBON OR OTHER WHISKEY

1½ TABLESPOONS BROWN SUGAR

½ TEASPOON SALT

4 BONELESS CENTER-CUT
    PORK CHOPS

1 TABLESPOON CHOPPED FRESH SAGE,
    FOR GARNISH

1. Preheat the oven to 375°F.

2. Spray a large, oven-safe skillet with nonstick cooking spray and place it in the oven to heat up.

3. Heat the olive oil in a small saucepan set over medium heat. When the oil is hot, stir in the pecans and cook, stirring frequently, until they are lightly browned and fragrant, 1 to 2 minutes.

4. Stir in the broth, bourbon, sugar, and salt, and bring to a simmer. Reduce the heat to medium-low and cook, stirring often, until the sauce thickens and reduces by about one-third, 6 to 8 minutes. Reduce the heat to low and keep the sauce warm.

5. Place the pork chops in the hot skillet and cook them in the oven for about 8 minutes, until they are nicely browned on the bottom. Turn the chops over and cook until they are browned on the other side and cooked through, 8 to 10 minutes more.

6. Serve the pork chops immediately, topped with the sauce and garnished with sage.

NUTRITIONAL INFORMATION PER SERVING: CALORIES 246 TOTAL FAT 10.3G SATURATED FAT 2.3G
TRANS FAT 0.0G SODIUM 376MG TOTAL CARBOHYDRATES 4.6G SUGARS 3.7G PROTEIN 25.7G

Garlic-Oregano Pork Loin

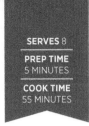
A pork loin takes only a few minutes to prepare before you put it in the oven, but it can feed a large number of people. A 2½-pound roast, for example, can feed up to eight. Serve it with mashed potatoes and glazed carrots or other root vegetables for a hearty Sunday supper.

1 (2½-POUND) BONELESS PORK LOIN

SALT

FRESHLY GROUND BLACK PEPPER

1 TABLESPOON MINCED GARLIC

2 TEASPOONS DRIED OREGANO

1. Preheat the oven to 400°F.

2. Line a roasting pan with foil.

3. Trim the fat from the pork, if desired, leaving a layer of fat on top. Season the pork with salt and pepper.

4. Rub the garlic into the pork and sprinkle it with the oregano, then place it fat-side down in the roasting pan.

5. Roast the pork for 30 minutes, then turn it over and roast it for another 25 minutes, or until it reaches an internal temperature of 155°F.

6. Remove the loin to a cutting board and let it rest for 10 minutes before slicing.

NUTRITIONAL INFORMATION PER SERVING: CALORIES 411 TOTAL FAT 10.0G SATURATED FAT 3.4G TRANS FAT 0.1G SODIUM 201MG TOTAL CARBOHYDRATES 1.2G SUGARS 0.0G PROTEIN 74.4G

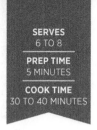

SERVES
6 TO 8

PREP TIME
5 MINUTES

COOK TIME
30 TO 40 MINUTES

Easy Roast Beef

Roast beef is classic comfort food. It may take a little longer to cook than some other recipes, but the preparation is simple and it is well worth the wait. Serve it with a dollop of prepared horseradish and roasted potatoes for a classic presentation.

1 (2½- TO 3-POUND) BONELESS BEEF
    ROUND ROAST

SALT

FRESHLY GROUND BLACK PEPPER

2 TABLESPOONS EXTRA-VIRGIN
    OLIVE OIL

2 TABLESPOONS DIJON MUSTARD

1 TABLESPOON MINCED GARLIC

1 TEASPOON BALSAMIC VINEGAR

1. Preheat the oven to 475°F.

2. Season the roast with salt and pepper.

3. Heat the olive oil in a skillet over medium-high heat and add the roast. Sear the roast for 2 minutes on each side, or until it is lightly browned.

4. Transfer the beef to a roasting pan.

5. In a small bowl, whisk together the mustard, garlic, and vinegar and rub the mixture into the roast.

6. Roast the beef for 25 to 30 minutes (to an internal temperature of 125°F) for medium-rare or for 30 to 35 minutes (to an internal temperature of 130°F) for medium.

7. Remove the roast to a cutting board and let it rest for 10 minutes before carving.

NUTRITIONAL INFORMATION PER SERVING: CALORIES 528 TOTAL FAT 37.1G SATURATED FAT 12.7G
TRANS FAT 0.0G SODIUM 197MG TOTAL CARBOHYDRATES 0.8G SUGARS 0.0G PROTEIN 44.5G

Classic Sloppy Joes

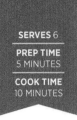

SERVES 6

PREP TIME
5 MINUTES

COOK TIME
10 MINUTES

Sloppy joes are a quick and satisfying weeknight supper. This version replaces wheat flour with gluten-free all-purpose flour (homemade recipe on page 32). Serve it atop your favorite gluten-free hamburger buns. The sauce will soak into the bread, and you won't even notice that they're not wheat hamburger buns.

1 POUND GROUND BEEF

1 CUP KETCHUP

1 CUP FINELY CHOPPED CELERY

½ CUP DICED ONION

1 TABLESPOON BROWN SUGAR

1 TABLESPOON WHITE VINEGAR

½ TEASPOON DRY MUSTARD POWDER

2 TABLESPOONS GLUTEN-FREE
    ALL-PURPOSE FLOUR, PLUS MORE
    IF NEEDED

6 GLUTEN-FREE HAMBURGER BUNS

1. Heat a skillet over medium heat. Add the beef and cook, stirring, until thoroughly browned, about 5 minutes. Drain off the excess fat and return the pan to the heat.

2. Add the ketchup, celery, onion, brown sugar, vinegar, and mustard to the skillet, and stir to mix well. Add the flour, sprinkling it over the beef mixture, and stir to combine.

3. Cook, stirring frequently, until the mixture is bubbling and thick, 4 to 5 minutes. Add additional flour if needed.

4. To serve, place the opened buns onto serving plates and spoon the beef mixture over the bottom halves. Place the top of the bun on top of the beef mixture and enjoy.

NUTRITIONAL INFORMATION PER SERVING: CALORIES 454   TOTAL FAT 11.0G   SATURATED FAT 2.3G
TRANS FAT 0.0G   **SODIUM** 822MG   **TOTAL CARBOHYDRATES** 61.8G   **SUGARS** 15.4G   **PROTEIN** 29.9G

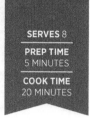

Skillet-Browned Meatballs

These would pair perfectly with cooked gluten-free pasta and your favorite tomato sauce. Top with a fresh grating of Parmesan cheese, and you have an old-school, deeply satisfying plate of spaghetti and meatballs.

Time-saving tip Standing over a skillet cooking meatballs is time-consuming, especially if you're making a large batch. Browning the meatballs in the oven frees you up to do other things while they cook. Preheat the oven to 400°F. Place the meatballs on a baking sheet sprayed with nonstick cooking spray. Spritz a bit of nonstick cooking spray on top of the meatballs. Bake the meatballs for about 20 minutes, turning them once after 10 minutes, until the meatballs are cooked through and nicely browned on the outside.

2 POUNDS LEAN GROUND BEEF

1 TABLESPOON MINCED GARLIC

2 EGGS, LIGHTLY BEATEN

1 CUP FRESHLY GRATED ROMANO CHEESE

¼ CUP CHOPPED FRESH
    FLAT-LEAF PARSLEY

1 TEASPOON DRIED OREGANO

SALT

FRESHLY GROUND BLACK PEPPER

EXTRA-VIRGIN OLIVE OIL, FOR
    COOKING

1. In a medium bowl, combine the beef, garlic, eggs, Romano cheese, parsley, and oregano. Season the mixture with salt and pepper. Blend the ingredients well by hand or with a wooden spoon.

2. Shape the beef mixture into 1½-inch meatballs and put them on a plate.

3. Grease a heavy skillet with olive oil and heat over medium heat.

4. Add about half the meatballs to the skillet. Cook the meatballs for 8 minutes or so, turning frequently, until they are cooked through. Transfer the meatballs to a plate in a warm oven to keep hot. Repeat with the remaining meatballs.

5. Serve the meatballs hot.

NUTRITIONAL INFORMATION PER SERVING: CALORIES 313 TOTAL FAT 14.7G SATURATED FAT 6.3G
TRANS FAT 0.0G SODIUM 324MG TOTAL CARBOHYDRATES 1.3G SUGARS 0.0G PROTEIN 41.6G

Homemade Meatloaf

SERVES 4

PREP TIME
5 MINUTES

COOK TIME
35 MINUTES

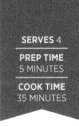

Meatloaf is a staple of family dinners, and this recipe is made with gluten-free oats instead of flour so it is safe for the whole family. Served alongside mashed potatoes and steamed or roasted vegetables, it's pretty much a perfect meal. The leftovers are great in sandwiches, too. Try slices of meatloaf on Basic Sandwich Bread (page 36) for lunch.

1 POUND LEAN GROUND BEEF

½ CUP GLUTEN-FREE ROLLED OATS

5 TABLESPOONS KETCHUP

¼ CUP MINCED YELLOW ONION

1 EGG, LIGHTLY BEATEN

1 TEASPOON SALT

½ TEASPOON DRIED OREGANO

½ TEASPOON FRESHLY GROUND
   BLACK PEPPER

1. Preheat the oven to 375°F.

2. Line a baking pan with foil.

3. In a medium bowl, combine the beef, oats, ketchup, onion, egg, salt, oregano, and pepper, and stir well to combine.

4. Shape the mixture into a loaf by hand and then place it into in the middle of the baking pan.

5. Bake the meatloaf for 35 minutes, or until the meatloaf is cooked through.

6. Let the meatloaf sit for 5 minutes, then slice it to serve.

NUTRITIONAL INFORMATION PER SERVING: CALORIES 294 TOTAL FAT 9.1G SATURATED FAT 3.0G
TRANS FAT 0.0G SODIUM 880MG TOTAL CARBOHYDRATES 13.8G SUGARS 4.7G PROTEIN 38.0G

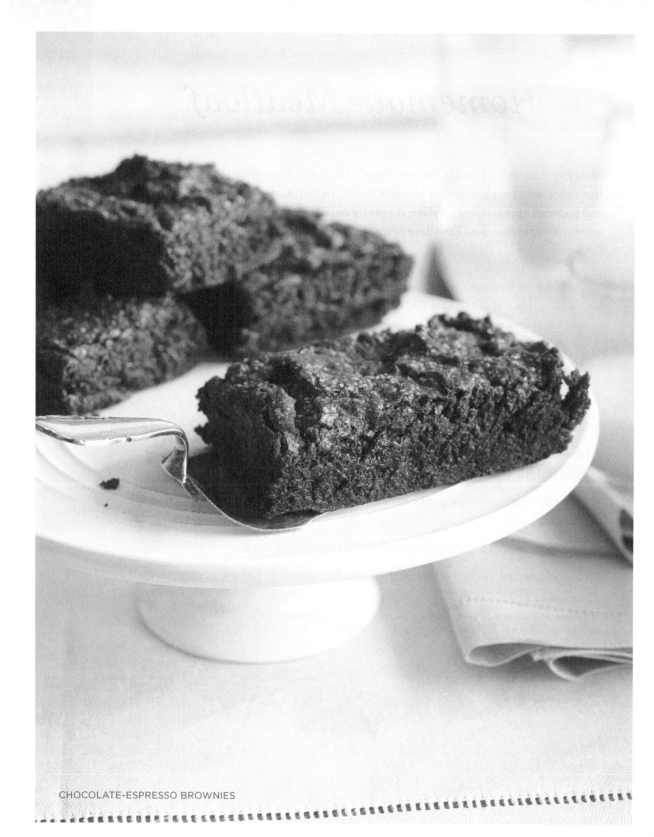

CHOCOLATE-ESPRESSO BROWNIES

11

Desserts

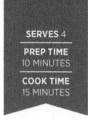
Cinnamon-Raisin Baked Apples

Baked apples, filled to bursting with raisins and honey, taste like apple pie without the crust. If you are in the mood for a more decadent dessert, top them with vanilla ice cream or a dollop of lightly sweetened whipped cream.

4 APPLES

½ CUP RAISINS

2½ TABLESPOONS HONEY

1 TABLESPOON BROWN SUGAR

1 TEASPOON GROUND CINNAMON

1 CUP UNSWEETENED APPLE JUICE

1. Preheat the oven to 350°F.

2. Use a sharp knife to cut about 1 inch off the tops of the apples and set the tops aside. Carefully scoop the cores from the apples and discard.

3. In a small bowl, stir together the raisins, honey, brown sugar, and cinnamon.

4. Arrange the apples in a small glass baking dish. Spoon the raisin mixture into the apples and place the tops back on.

5. Pour the apple juice into the pan around the apples.

6. Bake the apples for 15 minutes, or until they are very tender.

7. Serve the apples warm, with the pan juices spooned over them.

NUTRITIONAL INFORMATION PER SERVING: CALORIES 228 TOTAL FAT 0.2G SATURATED FAT 0.0G TRANS FAT 0.0G SODIUM 7MG TOTAL CARBOHYDRATES 60.2G SUGARS 49.4G PROTEIN 0.7G

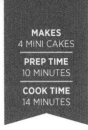

MAKES
4 MINI CAKES

PREP TIME
10 MINUTES

COOK TIME
14 MINUTES

Molten Chocolate Mini Cakes

Popularized by chichi restaurants, these simple, elegant, divinely rich chocolate cakes couldn't be easier to make. Made in individual-sized servings and literally oozing chocolatey goodness, they are special enough to serve for a special meal, but easy enough to make any time you please. Top with a dollop of whipped cream or whipped coconut cream, if desired.

4 OUNCES SEMI-SWEET CHOCOLATE,
    FINELY CHOPPED
½ CUP UNSALTED BUTTER
1 CUP POWDERED SUGAR
2 EGGS, LIGHTLY BEATEN
2 EGG YOLKS

6 TABLESPOONS GLUTEN-FREE
    ALL-PURPOSE FLOUR
POWDERED SUGAR, FOR GARNISH
    (OPTIONAL)
BERRIES, FOR GARNISH (OPTIONAL)

1. Preheat the oven to 425°F, coat four 4-ounce ramekins or custard cups with butter, and place them place on a baking sheet.

2. In the top of a double boiler set over simmering water, combine the butter and chocolate and cook, stirring, until the butter is melted and the chocolate is mostly melted. Remove from the heat and stir until smooth.

3. Scoop the batter into the prepared ramekins, dividing equally. Slide the baking sheet with the filled ramekins on it into the preheated oven and bake for 14 minutes. Remove from the oven and let cool for 1 minute. Run a knife around the edge of the cakes to loosen them and then invert the ramekins onto serving plates. Sprinkle with powdered sugar and top with a handful of berries, if desired. Serve warm.

NUTRITIONAL INFORMATION PER SERVING: CALORIES 553   TOTAL FAT 34.5G   SATURATED FAT 19.4G
TRANS FAT 0.0G   SODIUM 321MG   TOTAL CARBOHYDRATES 57.5G   SUGARS 41.8G   PROTEIN 6.4G

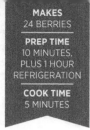

MAKES
24 BERRIES

PREP TIME
10 MINUTES,
PLUS 1 HOUR
REFRIGERATION

COOK TIME
5 MINUTES

Chocolate-Covered Strawberries

Chocolate-covered strawberries don't have to be reserved for special occasions. With this simple recipe, you make them quickly and can keep them in the refrigerator to enjoy whenever you please. That said, you might not want to make them all the time. You need something to surprise your sweetie with on Valentine's Day, after all.

Cooking tip Make sure your strawberries are very dry before you begin dipping them. Water on the berries will cause your chocolate to clump into a thick paste, destroying its smooth texture.

24 WHOLE LARGE STRAWBERRIES

2 CUPS SEMISWEET CHOCOLATE CHIPS

½ TABLESPOON COCONUT OIL

1. Line a baking sheet with parchment paper.

2. Carefully remove the leaves from the strawberries by hand, and use the stems to hold the strawberries.

3. Place the chocolate chips in the top of a double boiler set over simmering water. If you do not have a double broiler, you can create your own by setting a large, stainless steel bowl over a saucepot with simmering water. Cook, stirring frequently, until the chocolate is completely melted and smooth, about 5 minutes.

4. Stir the coconut oil into the warm chocolate to melt it and to thin the chocolate.

5. Dip the strawberries in the chocolate and place them on the baking sheet about ½ inch to 1 inch apart.

6. Place the baking sheet in the refrigerator until the chocolate hardens, about 1 hour. Serve cold.

7. Store the strawberries in the refrigerator for up to 2 days.

NUTRITIONAL INFORMATION PER STRAWBERRY: CALORIES 129   TOTAL FAT 5.9G   SATURATED FAT 3.6G   TRANS FAT 0.0G   SODIUM 1MG   TOTAL CARBOHYDRATES 20.0G   SUGARS 14.2G   PROTEIN 0.7G

Chocolate-Peppermint Bark

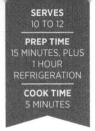

SERVES
10 TO 12

PREP TIME
15 MINUTES, PLUS
1 HOUR
REFRIGERATION

COOK TIME
5 MINUTES

Chocolate and peppermint are two flavors that were simply meant to be together. This is a lovely treat to have around for a sweet after-dinner nibble. Make a large batch and wrap up portions in pretty packaging to give away as holiday gifts.

Ingredient tip You could make this recipe with milk chocolate chips or bittersweet chocolate chips. For a pretty effect, try layering dark and white chocolate. Follow the directions for the semisweet chips, but before adding the peppermint candy, melt the same quantity of white chocolate chips and smooth that over the top of the dark chocolate. Then add the peppermint candy and proceed with the recipe.

2 CUPS SEMISWEET CHOCOLATE CHIPS

¼ TEASPOON PEPPERMINT EXTRACT

1¼ CUPS CRUSHED
PEPPERMINT CANDIES

1. Line a large rimmed baking sheet with foil and set aside.

2. Place the chocolate chips in the top of a double boiler set over simmering water. If you do not have a double broiler, you can create your own by setting a large, stainless steel bowl over a saucepot with simmering water. Cook, stirring frequently, until the chocolate is completely melted and smooth, about 5 minutes.

3. Whisk in the peppermint extract.

4. Pour the chocolate onto the baking sheet and spread evenly.

5. Sprinkle the chocolate immediately with the crushed peppermint candies and gently press them into the chocolate.

6. Chill the bark in the refrigerator until the chocolate is set, about 1 hour.

7. Break the bark into pieces by hand and serve cold.

8. Store the bark in an airtight container for up to 2 weeks.

NUTRITIONAL INFORMATION PER SERVING: CALORIES 260 TOTAL FAT 12.8G SATURATED FAT 8.0G
TRANS FAT 0.0G SODIUM 0MG TOTAL CARBOHYDRATES 38.4G SUGARS 31.2G PROTEIN 0.0G

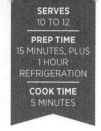

SERVES
10 TO 12

PREP TIME
15 MINUTES, PLUS
1 HOUR
REFRIGERATION

COOK TIME
5 MINUTES

White and Dark Chocolate Walnut Bark

Studded with white chocolate chips and walnut chunks, this chocolate treat is as pretty as it is delicious. It's another easy dessert to whip up and have around to satisfy your sweet tooth. And wrapped up with pretty ribbon, it makes a lovely gift, too.

2 CUPS SEMISWEET
CHOCOLATE CHIPS

½ TEASPOON VANILLA EXTRACT

1 CUP WHITE CHOCOLATE
BAKING CHIPS

½ CUP CHOPPED WALNUTS

1. Line a large rimmed baking sheet with foil and set aside.

2. Place the chocolate chips in the top of a double boiler set over simmering water. If you do not have a double broiler, you can create your own by setting a large, stainless steel bowl over a saucepot with simmering water. Cook, stirring frequently, until the chocolate is completely melted and smooth, about 5 minutes.

3. Whisk in the vanilla extract.

4. Pour the chocolate onto the baking sheet and spread out evenly.

5. Sprinkle the chocolate with the white chocolate baking chips and let it sit for a few minutes until the white chocolate melts. Smooth the white chocolate into an even layer, being careful not to mix it into the dark chocolate.

6. Add the walnuts, pressing them gently into the bark.

7. Chill the bark in the refrigerator until the chocolate is set, about 1 hour.

8. Break the bark into pieces by hand.

9. Store the bark in an airtight container in a cool place for up to 2 weeks.

NUTRITIONAL INFORMATION PER SERVING: CALORIES 332 TOTAL FAT 20.5G SATURATED FAT 11.2G
TRANS FAT 0.0G SODIUM 15MG TOTAL CARBOHYDRATES 38.3G SUGARS 31.4G PROTEIN 2.5G

Lemon-Lime Sorbet

SERVES
8 TO 10

PREP TIME
15 MINUTES, PLUS
2 TO 3 HOURS
FREEZING TIME

COOK TIME
7 MINUTES

Made from fruit and sugar, sorbet is a delicious and refreshing fat-free alternative to ice cream. This particular recipe combines the tart flavors of lemon and lime with the rich sweetness of honey for a particularly tasty and guilt-free treat.

Cooking tip Homemade sorbet sometimes becomes too icy or freezes rock solid. To prevent this, give your sorbet a shot of booze. Alcohol has a very high freezing point, so it keeps the texture of your sorbet soft. You don't need much. Just a tablespoon or so is enough to do the trick. Try a neutral-tasting alcohol like vodka, unless you want a distinctly cocktail-flavored dessert.

1½ CUPS WATER

¼ CUP HONEY

½ CUP FRESHLY SQUEEZED
    LEMON JUICE

¾ CUP FRESHLY SQUEEZED LIME JUICE

2 TABLESPOONS LEMON ZEST

1 TABLESPOON LIME ZEST

1. In a small saucepan over medium-low heat, whisk together the water, honey, lemon juice, and lime juice.

2. Cook the mixture, stirring well, until the honey melts, about 5 minutes.

3. Stir in the lemon zest and lime zest and cook, stirring often, for 2 minutes.

4. Remove the mixture from the heat and strain it through a mesh sieve into a shallow dish. Discard the solids.

5. Freeze the sorbet in a shallow dish until it is solid, 2 to 3 hours.

6. Just before serving the sorbet, break it into pieces and blend it smooth in a food processor or blender.

7. Store the sorbet in a freezer-proof container, with a piece of plastic wrap pressed to the surface, in the freezer for 1 to 2 months.

NUTRITIONAL INFORMATION PER SERVING: CALORIES 30 TOTAL FAT 0.1G SATURATED FAT 0.0G TRANS FAT 0.0G SODIUM 4MG TOTAL CARBOHYDRATES 7.6G SUGARS 7.3G PROTEIN 0.2G

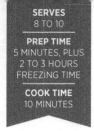

SERVES
8 TO 10

PREP TIME
5 MINUTES, PLUS
2 TO 3 HOURS
FREEZING TIME

COOK TIME
10 MINUTES

Raspberry Sorbet

Raspberries are incredibly rich in antioxidants. A single cup contains more than 50 percent of your daily recommended dose of vitamin C. Here they're combined with rich, sweet honey and a dash of tart lemon juice, then frozen into an irresistible, scoopable dessert.

1½ CUPS WATER

¼ CUP HONEY

2 TABLESPOONS FRESHLY SQUEEZED LEMON JUICE

3 CUPS FRESH RASPBERRIES

1. In a medium saucepan over medium-low heat, whisk together the water, honey, and lemon juice.

2. Cook the mixture, stirring well, until the honey melts, about 5 minutes.

3. Add the raspberries and cook for an additional 5 minutes, stirring, until the berries are steaming.

4. Remove the saucepan from the heat and strain the berry mixture through a mesh sieve into a shallow dish. Discard the solids.

5. Freeze the sorbet in a shallow pan, 2 to 3 hours.

6. Just before serving the sorbet, break it into pieces and blend it smooth in a food processor or blender.

7. Store the sorbet in a freezer-proof container, with a piece of plastic wrap pressed to the surface, in the freezer for 1 to 2 months.

NUTRITIONAL INFORMATION PER SERVING: **CALORIES** 57 **TOTAL FAT** 0.3G **SATURATED FAT** 0.0G
TRANS FAT 0.0G **SODIUM** 3MG **TOTAL CARBOHYDRATES** 14.3G **SUGARS** 10.8G **PROTEIN** 0.6G

SERVES 6
PREP TIME
15 MINUTES, PLUS
2 TO 3 HOURS
FREEZING TIME
COOK TIME
5 MINUTES

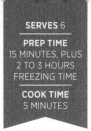

Cappuccino Chip Frozen Yogurt

This cool and creamy dessert has a subtle coffee flavor and a smattering of mini chocolate chips. Evaporated milk (not to be confused with sweetened condensed milk) provides a rich, creamy flavor without the fat of heavy cream.

Time-saving tip Use a microwave to cut the prep time of this recipe. Combine the milk and sugar in a medium glass bowl, instead of a saucepan, and heat it in the microwave at 50 percent power for 1 minute. Stir to see if the sugar is melted. If not, heat it for 15 seconds more and stir again. Repeat until the sugar is melted. Remove the mixture from the microwave and whisk until smooth.

1 (12-OUNCE) CAN EVAPORATED MILK

¾ CUP SUPERFINE SUGAR

2 TEASPOONS CORNSTARCH

½ TEASPOON VANILLA EXTRACT

1 CUP PLAIN NONFAT YOGURT

¼ CUP BREWED COFFEE, COOLED

¾ CUP MINI CHOCOLATE CHIPS

1. In a small saucepan over medium heat, combine the evaporated milk and sugar and cook, stirring frequently, until the sugar melts, about 5 minutes.

2. Whisk in the cornstarch and vanilla and let it sit for 5 minutes.

3. Stir in the yogurt and cooled coffee, whisking until smooth. Fold in the chocolate chips.

4. Pour the mixture into an ice cream maker and freeze it according to the manufacturer's directions.

5. If you don't have an ice cream maker, pour it into a freezer-proof container and freeze it until it is solid, 2 to 3 hours. Thaw the yogurt for 10 minutes to soften it before serving.

6. Store the yogurt in a freezer-proof container in the freezer for 1 to 2 months.

NUTRITIONAL INFORMATION PER SERVING: CALORIES 316 TOTAL FAT 11.0G SATURATED FAT 7.4G
TRANS FAT 0.0G **SODIUM** 106MG **TOTAL CARBOHYDRATES** 46.9G **SUGARS** 44.4G **PROTEIN** 7.8G

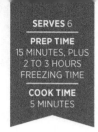
SERVES 6

PREP TIME
15 MINUTES, PLUS
2 TO 3 HOURS
FREEZING TIME

COOK TIME
5 MINUTES

Almond Butter Frozen Yogurt

Almond butter, though less commonly used than peanut butter, is just as creamy and flavorful, particularly in this recipe. Combined with evaporated milk and nonfat yogurt, it blends up into a rich, creamy frozen dessert that's as delicious as any ice cream.

1 (12-OUNCE) CAN EVAPORATED MILK

¾ CUP SUPERFINE SUGAR

½ CUP ALMOND BUTTER

2 TEASPOONS CORNSTARCH

1 TEASPOON VANILLA EXTRACT

1 CUP PLAIN NONFAT YOGURT

1. In a medium saucepan set over medium heat, combine the milk, sugar, and almond butter. Cook, whisking constantly, until the sugar dissolves and the mixture is smooth, about 5 minutes. Lower the heat if necessary so that the mixture doesn't boil.

2. Whisk in the cornstarch and vanilla extract and let it sit for 5 minutes.

3. Add the yogurt, whisking until smooth.

4. Pour the mixture into an ice cream maker and freeze it according to the manufacturer's directions.

5. If you don't have an ice cream maker, pour the mixture into a freezer-proof container and freeze it until it is solid, 2 to 3 hours. Thaw the yogurt for 10 minutes to soften it before serving.

6. Store the yogurt in a freezer-proof container in the freezer for 1 to 2 months.

NUTRITIONAL INFORMATION PER SERVING: CALORIES 336   TOTAL FAT 16.6G   SATURATED FAT 4.1G
TRANS FAT 0.0G   **SODIUM** 89MG   **TOTAL CARBOHYDRATES** 38.1G   **SUGARS** 33.6G   **PROTEIN** 10.6G

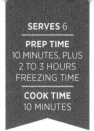

SERVES 6

PREP TIME
10 MINUTES, PLUS
2 TO 3 HOURS
FREEZING TIME

COOK TIME
10 MINUTES

Blueberry Swirl Frozen Yogurt

Blueberries are always at their best when they are in season. So while blueberries give an especially dramatic visual effect to this dessert, feel free to substitute other berries, such as strawberries or raspberries, according to what's freshest and most flavorful in your market.

Ingredient tip Fresh blueberries are nice in this dessert, but let's face it: The whole thing is being frozen anyway, so don't hesitate to substitute frozen blueberries in a pinch.

1 (12-OUNCE) CAN EVAPORATED MILK

¾ CUP SUPERFINE SUGAR

1 CUP FRESH BLUEBERRIES

2 TABLESPOONS FRESHLY SQUEEZED
    LEMON JUICE

2 TEASPOONS CORNSTARCH

1 TEASPOON VANILLA EXTRACT

1 CUP PLAIN NONFAT YOGURT

1. In a double boiler over medium-low heat, combine the evaporated milk and sugar. If you do not have a double broiler, you can create your own by setting a large, stainless steel bowl over a saucepot with simmering water. Stir until the sugar melts, about 2 minutes.

2. Add the blueberries and gently stir to combine. Cook until the berries just begin to soften, about 5 minutes.

3. Stir in the lemon juice, cornstarch, and vanilla, then remove the mixture from the heat.

4. Stir in the yogurt, until smooth.

5. Pour the mixture into an ice cream maker and freeze it according to the manufacturer's directions.

continued ▶

Blueberry Swirl Frozen Yogurt *continued*

6. If you don't have an ice cream maker, pour the mixture into a freezer-proof container and freeze it until it is solid, 2 to 3 hours. Thaw the yogurt for 10 minutes to soften it before serving.

7. Store the yogurt in the freezer in a freezer-proof container for 1 to 2 months.

NUTRITIONAL INFORMATION PER SERVING: CALORIES 219   TOTAL FAT 4.9G   SATURATED FAT 3.1G   TRANS FAT 0.0G
SODIUM 90MG   TOTAL CARBOHYDRATES 38.1G   SUGARS 36.2G   PROTEIN 6.4G

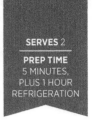

Chocolate Chia Seed Pudding

Chia seeds aren't just a novelty product anymore. They are the new superfood. Rich in dietary fiber and antioxidants, they also have the unique characteristic of soaking up liquid to form a pudding-like gel, making them a popular substitute for wheat-based thickeners, eggs, and dairy in puddings and other desserts.

1½ CUPS FAT-FREE MILK

¼ CUP CHIA SEEDS

3 TABLESPOONS UNSWEETENED COCOA POWDER

1 TABLESPOON HONEY

1. In a medium bowl, whisk together the milk, chia seeds, cocoa, and honey, until smooth.

2. Cover and chill the pudding in the refrigerator for about 1 hour, or until thickened.

3. Serve the pudding cold in individual dessert glasses.

NUTRITIONAL INFORMATION PER SERVING: CALORIES 176 TOTAL FAT 6.1G SATURATED FAT 1.0G
TRANS FAT 0.0G **SODIUM** 100MG **TOTAL CARBOHYDRATES** 28.0G **SUGARS** 17.8G **PROTEIN** 10.6G

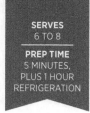

SERVES
6 TO 8

PREP TIME
5 MINUTES,
PLUS 1 HOUR
REFRIGERATION

Dairy-Free Chocolate Mousse

Heart-healthy avocado is the rich secret ingredient in this delicate honey-sweetened mousse. Try it the next time you are in the mood for something sweet but want it to be healthy. Be sure to chill the mousse very well before serving, or the avocado may overpower the other flavors.

3 AVOCADOS, PEELED, PITTED, AND
    CHOPPED
½ CUP UNSWEETENED COCOA POWDER

3 TABLESPOONS HONEY
1 TABLESPOON VANILLA EXTRACT
PINCH SALT

1. Place the avocado in a food processor or blender and blend until smooth.

2. Add the cocoa, honey, vanilla, and salt, and blend until thick and creamy.

3. Chill the mousse in the refrigerator until it thickens, about 1 hour.

4. Spoon the mousse into individual dessert glasses to serve.

NUTRITIONAL INFORMATION PER SERVING: CALORIES 260   TOTAL FAT 20.6G   SATURATED FAT 4.7G
TRANS FAT 0.0G   SODIUM 35MG   TOTAL CARBOHYDRATES 21.4G   SUGARS 9.5G   PROTEIN 3.3G

Chocolate Chip Cookies

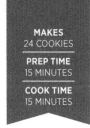

MAKES
24 COOKIES

PREP TIME
15 MINUTES

COOK TIME
15 MINUTES

Chocolate chip cookies are a staple of a happy childhood. Unhappy is the child who is denied them because of a gluten intolerance! The kids (and adults) in your household are sure to love this version—made with almond flour, which is rich in omega-3s and protein—and they won't even realize these cookies are gluten-free.

Time-saving tip Make a large batch of this cookie dough, form it into cookie-size balls, and freeze on a baking sheet. Bag the frozen balls, and then any time you want freshly baked cookies, just bake up as many or as few as you need. You may need to add an additional minute or two to the cooking time.

½ CUP COCONUT OIL, MELTED

½ CUP SUGAR

¼ CUP PACKED LIGHT BROWN SUGAR

2 EGGS, LIGHTLY BEATEN

1 TEASPOON VANILLA EXTRACT

PINCH SALT

3 CUPS ALMOND FLOUR

½ TEASPOON BAKING SODA

¾ CUP SEMISWEET CHOCOLATE CHIPS

1. Preheat the oven to 375°F.

2. Line a baking sheet with parchment paper.

3. In a large bowl, beat together the coconut oil, sugar, and light brown sugar.

4. Add the eggs and beat until smooth. Beat in the vanilla and salt.

5. In a medium bowl, combine the flour and baking soda.

6. Beat the flour mixture into the egg mixture in small batches until well combined. Fold in the chocolate chips.

7. Drop the batter in rounded tablespoons onto the prepared baking sheet, spacing the cookies about 1 inch apart.

8. Bake the cookies for 12 to 15 minutes, until they are lightly browned around the edges.

continued ▶

9. Cool the cookies for 3 minutes on the baking sheet, then transfer them to a wire rack to cool completely. Repeat until all the batter is used up.

10. If there are any cookies left over, store them in an airtight container at room temperature for up to 5 days.

NUTRITIONAL INFORMATION PER SERVING: CALORIES 123 TOTAL FAT 8.7G SATURATED FAT 5.4G TRANS FAT 0.0G
SODIUM 42MG TOTAL CARBOHYDRATES 11.5G SUGARS 9.8G PROTEIN 1.2G

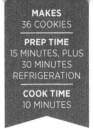

MAKES
36 COOKIES

PREP TIME
15 MINUTES, PLUS
30 MINUTES
REFRIGERATION

COOK TIME
10 MINUTES

Cranberry-Coconut Cookies

A blend of gluten-free flours gives these cookies that tender texture you want. Coconut oil contributes healthy monounsaturated fats and omega-3 fatty acids, and the unusual combination of coconut and cranberries gives these cookies a distinctive flavor.

2 CUPS RICE FLOUR

½ CUP COCONUT FLOUR

¼ CUP TAPIOCA STARCH

1 TEASPOON BAKING SODA

1 TEASPOON XANTHAN GUM

¼ TEASPOON SALT

½ CUP COCONUT OIL, MELTED

1 CUP PACKED LIGHT BROWN SUGAR

¼ CUP SUGAR

2 TABLESPOONS FAT-FREE MILK

2 EGGS

¾ CUP UNSWEETENED FLAKED
   COCONUT

¾ CUP DRIED CRANBERRIES

1. In a medium bowl, combine the rice flour, coconut flour, and tapioca starch. Add the baking soda, xanthan gum, and salt, and whisk gently to combine.

2. In a large bowl, beat together the coconut oil, brown sugar, sugar, and milk until smooth. Beat in the eggs.

3. Gradually stir the flour mixture into the egg mixture in small batches, until well combined.

4. Fold in the coconut and cranberries.

5. Turn the dough out onto a piece of plastic wrap. Gather it into a ball and wrap it with the plastic wrap. Chill the dough in the refrigerator for 30 minutes.

6. Preheat the oven to 375°F.

7. Line a baking sheet with parchment paper.

8. Pinch off tablespoon-size pieces of dough and roll them into balls. Arrange them on the prepared baking sheet, spacing them 1 inch apart. Gently flatten the cookies with a fork.

9. Bake the cookies for 8 to 10 minutes, until just lightly browned.

continued ▶

10. Cool the cookies in the pan for 3 to 4 minutes, then transfer them to a wire rack to cool completely. Repeat until all the batter is used up.

11. Store the cookies in an airtight container at room temperature for up to 5 days.

NUTRITIONAL INFORMATION PER SERVING: CALORIES 101 **TOTAL FAT** 4.1G **SATURATED FAT** 3.3G
TRANS FAT 0.0G **SODIUM** 154MG **TOTAL CARBOHYDRATES** 17.4G **SUGARS** 5.6G **PROTEIN** 1.4G

Walnut-Raisin Cookies

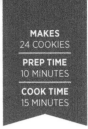

MAKES
24 COOKIES

PREP TIME
10 MINUTES

COOK TIME
15 MINUTES

When you bake cookies yourself, knowing for sure they are gluten-free is just one of many advantages. You can also make sure the ingredients are all-natural, can control the level of sweetness, and can load them up with whatever you like best. So go ahead and add more healthy walnuts and raisins, if that's how you like them.

½ CUP COCONUT OIL, MELTED

½ CUP SUGAR

¼ CUP PACKED LIGHT BROWN SUGAR

2 EGGS, LIGHTLY BEATEN

1 TEASPOON VANILLA EXTRACT

3 CUPS ALMOND FLOUR

½ TEASPOON BAKING SODA

PINCH SALT

½ CUP CHOPPED WALNUTS

¾ CUP RAISINS

1. Preheat the oven to 375°F.

2. Line a baking sheet with parchment paper.

3. In a large bowl, beat together the coconut oil, sugar, and brown sugar.

4. Add the eggs and beat until smooth. Beat in the vanilla.

5. In a medium bowl, combine the flour, baking soda, and salt.

6. Add the flour mixture to the egg mixture in small batches and beat until well combined. Fold in the walnuts and raisins.

7. Drop the batter by rounded tablespoons onto the prepared baking sheet, spacing the cookies about 1 inch apart.

8. Bake the cookies for 12 to 15 minutes, until they are lightly browned around the edges.

9. Cool the cookies for 3 minutes on the baking sheet, then transfer them to a wire rack to cool completely. Repeat until all the batter is used up.

10. Store the cookies in an airtight container at room temperature for up to 5 days.

NUTRITIONAL INFORMATION PER SERVING: CALORIES 107   TOTAL FAT 8.2G   SATURATED FAT 4.3G
TRANS FAT 0.0G   SODIUM 42MG   TOTAL CARBOHYDRATES 7.9G   SUGARS 6.7G   PROTEIN 1.9G

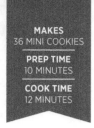

MAKES
36 MINI COOKIES

PREP TIME
10 MINUTES

COOK TIME
12 MINUTES

Mini Molasses Cookies

With the intense bite of cinnamon and ginger and the richness of molasses, these tiny cookies deliver big flavor. They are the perfect way to satisfy your sugar cravings without going off the gluten-free diet. And because they're small, you can eat twice as many of them, right?

¾ CUP PACKED BROWN SUGAR

½ CUP MOLASSES

¼ CUP COCONUT OIL, MELTED

6 EGGS, LIGHTLY BEATEN

¾ CUP COCONUT FLOUR

1 TEASPOON GROUND CINNAMON

½ TEASPOON GROUND GINGER

PINCH SALT

1. Preheat the oven to 400°F.

2. Line a baking sheet with parchment paper.

3. In a large bowl, whisk together the brown sugar, molasses, coconut oil, and eggs.

4. In a medium bowl, combine the flour, cinnamon, ginger, and salt.

5. Gradually beat the flour mixture into the egg mixture until smooth and combined.

6. Drop the batter by rounded tablespoons onto the prepared baking sheet.

7. Bake the cookies for 9 to 12 minutes, until they are just browned around the edges.

8. Cool the cookies for 5 minutes on the baking sheet, then transfer them to a wire rack to cool completely. Repeat until all the batter is used up.

9. Store the cookies in an airtight container at room temperature for up to 5 days.

NUTRITIONAL INFORMATION PER SERVING: CALORIES 59 TOTAL FAT 2.5G SATURATED FAT 1.6G
TRANS FAT 0.0G SODIUM 22MG TOTAL CARBOHYDRATES 7.8G SUGARS 5.7G PROTEIN 1.2G

Chocolate-Espresso Brownies

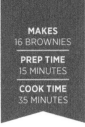

MAKES
16 BROWNIES

PREP TIME
15 MINUTES

COOK TIME
35 MINUTES

The slight bitter edge of freshly brewed espresso perfectly balances the sweet chocolate in these chewy brownies. Bake up a batch of these the next time you're asked to bring a dessert treat to a potluck or bake sale. They're sure to be a big hit.

NONSTICK COOKING SPRAY

¾ CUP COCONUT OIL

½ CUP UNSWEETENED COCOA POWDER

6 EGGS, LIGHTLY BEATEN

1 CUP HONEY

2 TABLESPOONS BREWED ESPRESSO, COOLED

1 TEASPOON VANILLA EXTRACT

½ CUP COCONUT FLOUR

⅛ TEASPOON SALT

1. Preheat the oven to 350°F.

2. Lightly grease an 8-by-8-inch glass baking dish with nonstick cooking spray.

3. In a small heavy saucepan over medium-low heat, combine the coconut oil and cocoa powder, stirring for 3 to 5 minutes, until the coconut oil melts. Remove the mixture from the heat and stir until smooth.

4. In a large bowl, combine the eggs, honey, espresso, and vanilla.

5. Add the coconut oil–cocoa mixture and beat until smooth. Stir in the coconut flour and salt until just combined.

6. Pour the mixture into the prepared baking dish and spread evenly.

7. Bake the brownies for 30 minutes, or until a toothpick inserted into the center of the brownies comes out clean.

8. Cool the brownies completely before cutting them into squares and serving.

9. Store the brownies in an airtight container at room temperature for up to 5 days.

NUTRITIONAL INFORMATION PER SERVING: CALORIES 170 TOTAL FAT 9.2G SATURATED FAT 6.7G
TRANS FAT 0.0G SODIUM 106MG TOTAL CARBOHYDRATES 21.1G SUGARS 17.9G PROTEIN 3.2G

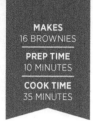

MAKES
16 BROWNIES

PREP TIME
10 MINUTES

COOK TIME
35 MINUTES

Chocolate–Peanut Butter Brownies

Rich, moist chocolate brownies are undeniably delicious, but add a dose of creamy peanut butter and they become pure heaven. This brownie recipe is sure to become one of your go-tos because everyone you serve them to will beg you to make them again and again.

Time-saving tip Use the microwave to melt the peanut butter to save time and cleanup. Place the peanut butter in a microwave-safe dish or small glass measuring cup at 15-second intervals on high heat until it melts. Stir until smooth.

NONSTICK COOKING SPRAY

¾ CUP COCONUT OIL

½ CUP UNSWEETENED COCOA
    POWDER

6 EGGS, LIGHTLY BEATEN

1 CUP HONEY

1 TEASPOON VANILLA EXTRACT

½ CUP COCONUT FLOUR

⅛ TEASPOON SALT

½ CUP SMOOTH PEANUT BUTTER

1. Preheat the oven to 350°F.

2. Lightly grease an 8-by-8-inch glass baking dish with nonstick cooking spray.

3. In a small heavy saucepan over medium-low heat, combine the coconut oil and cocoa powder, stirring for 3 to 5 minutes, until the coconut oil melts. Remove the mixture from the heat and stir until smooth.

4. In a large bowl, combine the eggs, honey, and vanilla extract.

5. Add the coconut oil–cocoa mixture and beat until smooth. Stir in the coconut flour and salt until just combined.

6. Spoon the mixture into the prepared baking dish and spread evenly.

7. Place the peanut butter in the top of a double boiler set over simmering water and cook, stirring, until it is melted and smooth, about 2 minutes. If you do not have a double broiler, you can create your own by setting a large, stainless steel bowl over a saucepot with simmering water.

8. Drizzle the melted peanut butter over the chocolate batter and swirl it into the batter with a knife.

9. Bake the brownies for 30 minutes, or until a toothpick inserted in the center of the brownies comes out clean.

10. Cool the brownies completely before cutting them into squares and serving.

11. Store the brownies in an airtight container at room temperature for up to 5 days.

NUTRITIONAL INFORMATION PER SERVING: CALORIES 217 TOTAL FAT 13.3G SATURATED FAT 7.6G
TRANS FAT 0.0G SODIUM 33MG TOTAL CARBOHYDRATES 22.7G SUGARS 18.6G PROTEIN 5.2G

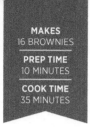

MAKES
16 BROWNIES

PREP TIME
10 MINUTES

COOK TIME
35 MINUTES

White and Dark Chocolate Brownies

If you can't decide between the sophistication of dark chocolate and the delicate sweetness of white chocolate, these brownies are the perfect solution. You get the deep richness of dark chocolate brownies lightened up with a sprinkling of white chocolate chips.

NONSTICK COOKING SPRAY

¾ CUP COCONUT OIL

½ CUP UNSWEETENED COCOA
    POWDER

6 EGGS, LIGHTLY BEATEN

1 CUP HONEY

1 TEASPOON VANILLA EXTRACT

½ CUP COCONUT FLOUR

⅛ TEASPOON SALT

¾ CUP WHITE CHOCOLATE
    BAKING CHIPS

1. Preheat the oven to 350°F.

2. Lightly grease an 8-by-8-inch glass baking dish with nonstick cooking spray.

3. In a small heavy saucepan over medium-low heat, combine the coconut oil and cocoa powder, stirring for 3 to 5 minutes, until the coconut oil melts. Remove the mixture from the heat and stir until smooth.

4. In a large bowl, combine the eggs, honey, and vanilla.

5. Add the coconut oil–cocoa mixture and beat until smooth. Stir in the coconut flour and salt until just combined.

6. Spoon the mixture into the prepared baking dish and spread evenly. Sprinkle the brownies with white chocolate chips.

7. Bake the brownies for 30 minutes, or until a toothpick inserted into the center of the brownies comes out clean.

8. Cool the brownies completely before cutting them into squares and serving. Store the brownies in an airtight container at room temperature for up to 5 days.

NUTRITIONAL INFORMATION PER SERVING: CALORIES 213 TOTAL FAT 11.7G SATURATED FAT 8.6G TRANS FAT 0.0G SODIUM 76MG TOTAL CARBOHYDRATES 26.6G SUGARS 23.4G PROTEIN 3.8G

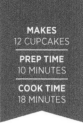

MAKES
12 CUPCAKES

PREP TIME
10 MINUTES

COOK TIME
18 MINUTES

Chocolate-Raspberry Cupcakes

No one can resist a fluffy chocolate cupcake, and this version is made extra special with the tart-sweet flavor of raspberries. Both raspberry jam and raspberry extract are added to the batter for a double dose of fruity flavor. These cupcakes are delicious just as they are, but they're even better topped with a spoonful of raspberry preserves and a dusting of confectioners' sugar.

3 CUPS ALMOND FLOUR

¼ CUP UNSWEETENED COCOA
    POWDER

½ TEASPOON BAKING SODA

⅛ TEASPOON SALT

½ CUP HONEY

¼ CUP COCONUT OIL, MELTED

3 EGGS, LIGHTLY BEATEN

2 TABLESPOONS RASPBERRY JAM

½ TEASPOON RASPBERRY EXTRACT

1. Preheat the oven to 350°F.

2. Line 12 cups of a standard muffin tin with paper liners.

3. In a medium bowl, combine the almond flour, cocoa powder, baking soda, and salt.

4. In a large bowl, beat together the honey, coconut oil, eggs, raspberry jam, and raspberry extract.

5. Whisk the dry ingredients into the wet ingredients until smooth.

6. Spoon the mixture into the muffin cups, filling each cup about two-thirds full.

7. Bake the cupcakes for 18 minutes, or until a toothpick inserted in the center of a cupcake comes out clean.

8. Cool the cupcakes for 5 minutes in the pan, then turn them out onto a wire rack to cool completely.

9. Store the cupcakes in an airtight container at room temperature for up to 2 days and in the refrigerator for up to 5 days.

NUTRITIONAL INFORMATION PER SERVING: CALORIES 151 TOTAL FAT 9.4G SATURATED FAT 4.7G
TRANS FAT 0.0G SODIUM 121MG TOTAL CARBOHYDRATES 16.5G SUGARS 13.6G PROTEIN 3.3G

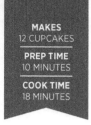

MAKES
12 CUPCAKES

PREP TIME
10 MINUTES

COOK TIME
18 MINUTES

Easy Vanilla Cupcakes

Sweet, moist, and full of rich vanilla flavor, white cupcakes are one of the most delightfully simple pleasures. These are a snap to throw together, making them the perfect recipe to reach for when you need a last-minute treat for a birthday party, bake sale, or other special occasion.

½ CUP COCONUT FLOUR

¼ TEASPOON BAKING SODA

⅛ TEASPOON SALT

½ CUP HONEY

½ CUP COCONUT OIL, MELTED

6 EGGS, LIGHTLY BEATEN

1 TEASPOON VANILLA EXTRACT

1. Preheat the oven to 350°F.

2. Line 12 cups of a standard muffin tin with paper liners.

3. In a small bowl, stir together the coconut flour, baking soda, and salt.

4. In a large bowl, beat together the honey, coconut oil, eggs, and vanilla.

5. Whisk the flour mixture into the egg mixture until smooth and well combined.

6. Spoon the batter into the muffin cups, filling each cup about two-thirds full.

7. Bake the cupcakes for 18 minutes, or until a toothpick inserted in the center of a cupcake comes out clean.

8. Cool the cupcakes in the pan for 5 minutes, then turn them out onto a wire rack to cool completely.

9. Store the cupcakes in an airtight container at room temperature for up to 2 days and in the refrigerator for up to 5 days.

NUTRITIONAL INFORMATION PER SERVING: CALORIES 174 TOTAL FAT 11.8G SATURATED FAT 8.7G
TRANS FAT 0.0G SODIUM 69MG TOTAL CARBOHYDRATES 14.5G SUGARS 12.1G PROTEIN 3.5G

Lemon-Coconut Cupcakes

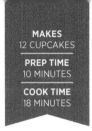

MAKES
12 CUPCAKES

PREP TIME
10 MINUTES

COOK TIME
18 MINUTES

These cupcakes are made with a triple dose of coconut—oil, flour, and flakes. A tart touch of lemon is a perfect balance. Whip some lemon zest and lemon juice with a little softened cream cheese for a quick frosting, if you like.

Ingredient tip For variety, substitute other citrus fruits for the lemon. Orange or lime would be especially nice here.

½ CUP COCONUT FLOUR

¼ TEASPOON BAKING SODA

⅛ TEASPOON SALT

½ CUP HONEY

½ CUP COCONUT OIL, MELTED

6 EGGS, LIGHTLY BEATEN

2 TABLESPOONS FRESHLY SQUEEZED
    LEMON JUICE

½ TEASPOON VANILLA EXTRACT

1 CUP UNSWEETENED FLAKED
    COCONUT

1. Preheat the oven to 350°F.

2. Line 12 cups of a standard muffin tin with paper liners.

3. In a small bowl, stir together the coconut flour, baking soda, and salt.

4. In a large bowl, beat together the honey, coconut oil, eggs, lemon juice, and vanilla.

5. Whisk the flour mixture into the egg mixture until smooth and well combined. Fold in the coconut.

6. Spoon the batter into the muffin cups, filling each cup about two-thirds full.

7. Bake the cupcakes for 18 minutes, or until a toothpick inserted in the center comes out clean.

8. Cool the cupcakes in the pan for 5 minutes, then turn them out onto a wire rack to cool completely.

9. Store the cupcakes in an airtight container at room temperature for up to 2 days and in the refrigerator for up to 5 days.

NUTRITIONAL INFORMATION PER SERVING: CALORIES 198   TOTAL FAT 14.0G   SATURATED FAT 10.7G
TRANS FAT 0.0G   **SODIUM** 71MG   **TOTAL CARBOHYDRATES** 15.6G   **SUGARS** 12.6G   **PROTEIN** 3.7G

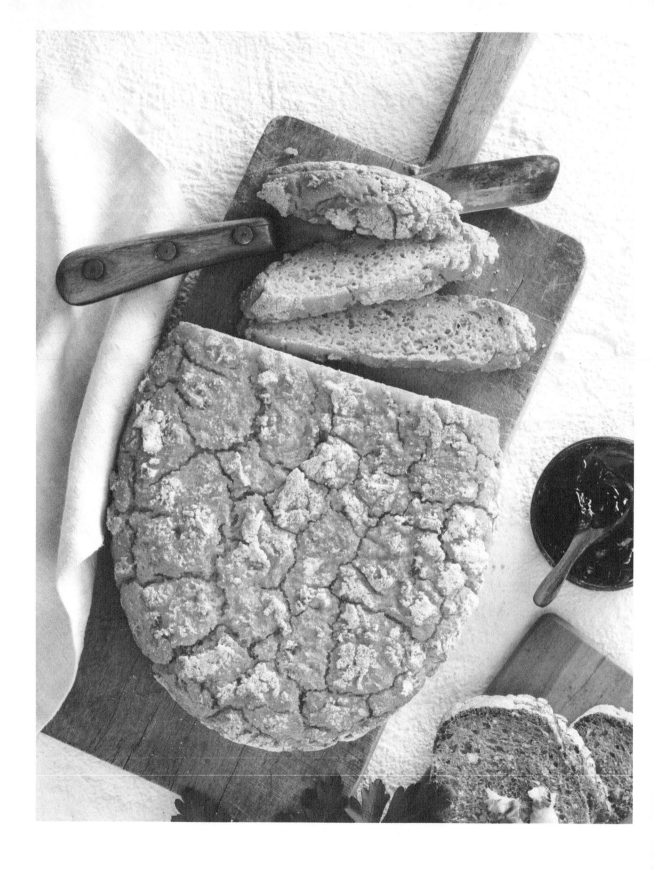

Gluten-Free Brands

More and more stores—from health food stores to mainstream supermarkets—are carrying gluten-free products. Here are some of the best brands of gluten-free products.

1-2-3 Gluten Free

This company offers gluten-free baking mixes, including cakes (both with and without sugar), cookies, and biscuits. They also offer a fortified gluten-free all-purpose flour mix.

You can find 1-2-3 Gluten Free products at Raley's, some Whole Foods, and online at 123GlutenFree.com.

Applegate

Applegate sells organic, all-natural meat products, including gluten-free bacon, frozen chicken nuggets and tenders, breakfast sausage, sausage links, chicken sausage, corn dogs, hot dogs, and deli meats.

You can find Applegate products at natural foods stores, including Trader Joe's and Whole Foods; at mainstream supermarkets, including Safeway, Raley's, and Target; and online at Applegate.com.

Authentic Foods

This company offers a wide range gluten-free flours and baking mixes—including brownies, cookies, cakes, pancakes and waffles, and even falafel mix.

Authentic Foods products are available at health food stores and natural foods stores, including Whole Foods, and online at AuthenticFoods.com.

Bob's Red Mill

Bob's Red Mill sells gluten-free active dry yeast, baking mixes, gluten-free flour alternatives (including grain flours, nut and seed meals, starches, and coconut flour), hot cereals, granola, guar and xanthan gums, soy protein, a gluten-free all-purpose flour blend, and various whole grains.

You can buy Bob's Red Mill products at natural foods stores, including Trader Joe's and Whole Foods; some mainstream supermarkets, including Lucky's; and online at BobsRedMill.com.

Enjoy Life Foods

Enjoy Life offers ready-made chips, cookies, breakfast cereals, granolas, snack bars, seed and fruit mixes, and baking chocolate that are not only gluten-free, but also free of the most common allergens, including dairy, peanuts, tree nuts, eggs, soy, fish, and shellfish.

You can buy Enjoy Life foods in many mainstream supermarkets, including Safeway, Raley's, and Target; in natural foods stores, including Whole Foods; and online at EnjoyLifeFoods.com.

Glutino

Glutino offers ready-made gluten-free foods, such as breads, crackers, pretzels, cookies, breakfast bars, pizzas, and complete frozen meals. They also offer baking mixes—for pancakes and waffles, brownies, cookies, cakes, muffins, pie crust, pizza crust, and cornbread— as well as an all-purpose flour mix.

You can find Glutino products at health food and natural foods stores, including Whole Foods, or online at Glutino.com.

Mary's Gone Crackers

Mary's Gone Crackers sells ready-made gluten-free crackers, cookies, pretzels, and breadcrumbs.

You can buy Mary's Gone Crackers products at natural foods stores, including Whole Foods; at Costco; and online at MarysGoneCrackers.com.

Namaste Foods

Namaste Foods sells gluten-free baking mixes, packaged macaroni and cheese, seasoning mixes, breading mixes, and instant soups.

Namaste Foods products are available at natural foods stores, such as Whole Foods; at mainstream supermarkets, including Albertson's and Publix; and online at NamasteFoods.com.

Pamela's Products

Pamela's Products offers baking mixes—breads, muffins, brownies, cookies, cakes, frostings, biscuits and scones, cornbread, pancakes and waffles, and pizza crust—as well as ready-made cookies and snack bars and an all-purpose gluten-free flour blend.

You can find Pamela's Products goods at health food and natural foods stores, including Whole Foods, or online at PamelasProducts.com.

Udi's Gluten Free

Udi's Gluten Free makes gluten-free breads, rolls, muffins, pizzas and pizza crusts, snack bars, granola, cookies, and brownies.

You can find Udi's Gluten Free products at natural foods stores, such as Whole Foods, or online at UdisGlutenFree.com.

The Dirty Dozen and the Clean Fifteen

EATING CLEAN

Each year, Environmental Working Group, an environmental organization based in the United States, publishes a list they call the "Dirty Dozen." These are the fruits and vegetables that, when conventionally grown using chemical pesticides and fertilizers, carry the highest residues. If organically grown isn't an option for you, simply avoid these fruits and vegetables altogether. The list is updated each year, but here is the most recent list (2013).

Similarly, the Environmental Working Group publishes a list of "The Clean Fifteen," fruits and vegetables that, even when conventionally grown, contain very low levels of chemical pesticide or fertilizer residue. These items are acceptable to purchase conventionally grown.

You might want to snap a photo of these two lists and keep them on your phone to reference while shopping. Or you can download the Environmental Working Groups app to your phone or tablet.

THE DIRTY DOZEN	THE CLEAN FIFTEEN
APPLE	ASPARAGUS
STRAWBERRY	AVOCADO
GRAPE	CABBAGE
CELERY	CANTALOUPE
PEACH	CORN
SPINACH	EGGPLANT
SWEET BELL PEPPER	GRAPEFRUIT
IMPORTED NECTARINE	KIWI
CUCUMBER	MANGO
CHERRY TOMATO	MUSHROOM
SNAP PEA	ONIONS
POTATO	PAPAYA
	PINEAPPLE
	SWEET PEAS (FROZEN)
	SWEET POTATO

UNIVERSAL

Conversion Charts

VOLUME EQUIVALENTS (LIQUID)		
U.S. STANDARD	U.S. STANDARD (OUNCES)	METRIC (APPROXIMATE)
2 TABLESPOONS	1 FL. OZ.	30 ML
¼ CUP	2 FL. OZ.	60 ML
½ CUP	4 FL. OZ.	120 ML
1 CUP	8 FL. OZ.	240 ML
1½ CUPS	12 FL. OZ.	355 ML
2 CUPS OR 1 PINT	16 FL. OZ.	475 ML
4 CUPS OR 1 QUART	32 FL. OZ.	1 L
1 GALLON	128 FL. OZ.	4 L

OVEN TEMPERATURES	
FAHRENHEIT (F)	CELSIUS (C) (APPROXIMATE)
250	120
300	150
325	165
350	180
375	190
400	200
425	220
450	230

VOLUME EQUIVALENTS (DRY)	
U.S. STANDARD	METRIC (APPROXIMATE)
⅛ TEASPOON	.5 ML
¼ TEASPOON	1 ML
½ TEASPOON	2 ML
¾ TEASPOON	4 ML
1 TEASPOON	5 ML
1 TABLESPOON	15 ML
¼ CUP	59 ML
⅓ CUP	79 ML
½ CUP	118 ML
⅔ CUP	156 ML
¾ CUP	177 ML
1 CUP	235 ML
2 CUPS OR 1 PINT	475 ML
3 CUPS	700 ML
4 CUPS OR 1 QUART	1 L
½ GALLON	2 L
1 GALLON	4 L

WEIGHT EQUIVALENTS	
U.S. STANDARD	METRIC (APPROXIMATE)
½ OUNCE	15 G
1 OUNCE	30 G
2 OUNCES	60 G
4 OUNCES	115 G
8 OUNCES	225 G
12 OUNCES	340 G
16 OUNCES OR 1 POUND	455 G

Resources

Celiac.com. "The Gluten-Free Diet 101—A Beginner's Guide to Going Gluten-Free." Accessed January 22, 2014. http://www.celiac.com/articles/22060/1/the-gluten-free-diet-101---a-beginners -guide-to-going-gluten-free/page1.html.

Celiac Disease Foundation. "What Is Celiac Disease?" Accessed April 18, 2014. http://celiac .org/celiac-disease/what-is-celiac-disease/.

Gluten-Free Living. "The Basic Diet (What I Can Eat)." Accessed January 1, 2014. http://www .glutenfreeliving.com/nutrition/the-basic-diet.

Harvard Medical School. "Considering a Gluten-Free Diet." Harvard Health Publications. April 2013. http://www.health.harvard.edu/newsletters/harvard_health_letter/2013/april /considering-a-gluten-free-diet.

Hyman, Mark. "Three Hidden Ways Wheat Makes You Fat." *Dr.Hyman.com.* Last modified January 25, 2013. http://drhyman.com/blog/2012/02/13/three-hidden-ways-wheat-makes-you -fat/#close.

Lapid, Nancy. "Gluten-Free Diet Guidelines for Celiac Disease." About.com, Celiac Disease & Gluten Sensitivity. Last updatedApril 10, 2014. http://celiacdisease.about.com/od /theglutenfreediet/a/GrainTable.htm.

Mayo Clinic Staff. "Gluten-Free Diet: What's Allowed, What's Not." Mayo Clinic. December 20, 2012. http://www.mayoclinic.org/gluten-free-diet/art-20048530.

National Foundation for Celiac Awareness. "Celiac Disease Facts & Figures." Accessed April 18, 2014. http://www.celiaccentral.org/celiac-disease/facts-and-figures/.

Storrs, Carina. "Will a Gluten-Free Diet Improve Your Health?" *Health.* Last modified April 5, 2011. http://www.health.com/health/article/0,,20479423,00.html.

Tallmadge, Katherine. "Should You Go Gluten-Free?" *Huffington Post.*July 8, 2013. http://www .huffingtonpost.com/2013/07/08/gluten-free-should-shouldnt_n_3561641.html#slide=624715.

University of Maryland Medical Center. "School of Medicine Researchers Identify Key Pathogenic Differences between Celiac Disease and Gluten Sensitivity." March 10, 2011. http://umm .edu/news-and-events/news-releases/2011/school-of-medicine-researchers-identify-key -pathogenic-differences-between-celiac-disease-and-gluten-sensitivity.

Verdu, Elena F., David Armstrong, and Joseph A. Murray. "Between Celiac Disease and Irritable Bowel Syndrome: The 'No Man's Land' of Gluten Sensitivity and IBS." *American Journal of Gastroenterology* 104 (June 2009): 1587–94. doi:10.1038/ajg.2009.188.

Whitehead, Erin. "12 Ways to Stick to Your Diet." *Woman's Day.* Accessed January 12, 2014. http://www.womansday.com/health-fitness/diet-weight-loss/12-ways-to-stick-to-your-diet-123115.

Zuckerbrot, Tanya. "Should You Go Gluten-Free?" *Prevention.* January 2013. http://www .prevention.com/food/healthy-eating-tips/benefits-and-downsides-gluten-free-eating.

IN 30 MINUTES

Recipe Index

IN 30 MINUTES

Index

CPSIA information can be obtained at www.ICGtesting.com
Printed in the USA
LVOW05*0227261114

415736LV00005B/16/P